A true back-owner's manual. Required reading for anyone ... back pain, has it now, or will have it.

> —Allen G. Zippin, MD, diplomate of the American Board of Neurological Surgery

Any book written to help people help themselves must contain technical details about how to do so—and this book is no exception. However, what distinguishes this book is that these gems are embedded in an account that personalizes Gerry Silverman to the reader. The stories of patients are presented with empathy and respect. The solutions to problems often enough originate in the application of some common sense plus some stretching and rubbing, so they are accessible to anyone. The book is easy, appropriate, convincingly honest, truly clinical—as well, I am sure, as an authoritative guide.

> —Harvey L. Lerner, MD, diplomate of the American Board of Internal Medicine

Healing is a spiritual as well as a physical challenge. Gerry Silverman has helped the work of healing with this wonderful book.

> —Rabbi Marc Gellman, Ph.D., senior rabbi of Temple Beth Torah in Melville, NY

YOUR Miraculous BACK

A

Step-by-Step

Guide to

Relieving

Neck &

Back Pain

GERALD M. SILVERMAN, DC

New Harbinger Publications, Inc.

Publisher's Note

This publication is designed to provide accurate and authoritative information in regard to the subject matter covered. It is sold with the understanding that the publisher is not engaged in rendering psychological, financial, legal, or other professional services. If expert assistance or counseling is needed, the services of a competent professional should be sought.

Distributed in Canada by Raincoast Books

Copyright © 2006 by Gerald Silverman
New Harbinger Publications, Inc.
5674 Shattuck Avenue
Oakland, CA 94609
www.newharbinger.com

Cover design by Amy Shoup
Text design by Michele Waters-Kermes
Illustrations by: Birck Cox Medical Illustration
Photography and Modeling by: Hampton Models
Acquired by Jess O'Brien
Edited by Jessica Beebe

Library of Congress Cataloging-in-Publication Data

Silverman, Gerald M.
   Your miraculous back : a step-by-step guide to relieving neck and back pain / Gerald
M. Silverman.
      p. cm.
   ISBN-13: 978-1-57224-452-8
   ISBN-10: 1-57224-452-6
   1. Backache—Alternative treatment. 2. Neck pain—Alternative treatment. 3.
Chiropractic. I. Title.
   RD771.B217S55 2006
   617.5'64062—dc22
                                   2006010776

08 07 06

10 9 8 7 6 5 4 3 2

For Randi, Ricki, and Ross

Contents

Introduction

Why another back pain book? With more books and products on the market for neck and back pain than for any other ailment, what could possibly be said or written that hasn't already been offered to the public? Yet with all the remedies and books available, and all the products you get to choose from, none have had a significant impact on the greatest nonlethal health epidemic to face this country. Every day, thousands of people get biological and psychological explanations of neck and back pain that are incorrect and don't adequately answer a few simple questions: Why is lower back pain so common in our society, and what makes it so difficult to treat? Why, in the absence of clearly defined physical findings, are so many patients overtreated, undertreated, or just plain mistreated? Despite all the advances in medicine and technology, why has the incidence, suffering, and cost of neck and lower back pain steadily increased over the last three decades? The answers will surprise you, help treat your pain, and surely change the way you think and feel about neck and lower back pain for the rest of your life. And that is exactly why there is a need for another neck and back pain book. There is a societal need to change attitudes, perceptions, treatments, and recommendations, because what's been done up to now just hasn't worked.

THE SOCIAL BURDEN OF BACK PAIN

The magnitude of neck and lower back pain in terms of suffering, medical costs, lost work time and wages, and disruption in the quality of life is staggering. Thirty-five million Americans are affected (Rizzo, Abbott, and Berger 1998), and the problem accounts for the country's greatest health care expenditure, at $60 billion annually (Frymoyer and Cats-Baril 1991). Neck and lower back pain are the second most common reason for medical office visits (just behind the common cold) and the number one cause of lost work time and disability claims (Agency for Health Care Policy and Research 1994). Each year, 83 million days of work are lost, and neck and back pain sufferers spend 200 million days in bed (Georgetown University Center on an Aging Society 2003). These patients spend almost two and a half times as much on health care as other patients, but those costs vary dramatically depending upon socioeconomic and demographic influences and not on the condition itself (Manek and MacGregor 2005). Lower back pain is the most common cause of inactivity in people under age forty-five (Agency for Health Care Policy and Research 1994). It's time we gave this epidemic our full attention. By doing so, we can dramatically reduce its grip on society.

If you're like most people, you've tried several therapies over the years and have probably received some temporary relief. You've also gotten several different diagnoses, various explanations, and conflicting opinions, some from medical professionals and many more from well-meaning friends. The only things that remain constant, however, are your confusion, frustration, and the reoccurring neck or lower back pain.

This book will offer you a closer look at the most basic causes of neck and lower back pain and provide some reassurance that with a little effort and determination, you can beat this problem once and for all.

IT'S UP TO YOU

Because wedging yourself into an uncomfortable chair and then not moving your neck is the last thing you want to do when you're in pain, I will be as brief and to the point as possible. Not everything in this book is agreed upon by all health professionals, and not everything will be right for every reader. You must find the combination of therapies that's right for you, and this book will help you do exactly that. If you leave your care to someone else—someone who has two hundred other patients to think about or someone whose understanding of back pain hasn't changed since medical school twenty years ago—here's what you're likely to get.

See a general practitioner, and he will probably prescribe pain medication and tell you the pain will go away. If it doesn't, he'll refer you to an orthopedist. Orthopedists most often prescribe anti-inflammatory medication and physical therapy and tell you the pain will go away. If it doesn't, they refer you to a neurologist, who will run a battery of tests and then repeat what the orthopedists have already said. Next up you have the surgeon, and if you make it to this point, she will undoubtedly repeat what the orthopedist and neurologist told you. If the pain still hasn't gone away, she'll want to operate.

Try the alternative care route, and you'll find that chiropractors will prescribe manipulation and adjustments. Acupuncturists will needle you. Massage therapists will rub a bit, and though massage feels good, it hasn't been shown to influence the outcome. Psychologists and psychiatrists—well, let's just say that blaming your parents, spouse, or boss won't make either of you feel better.

It is not my intent to bash respectable professionals, and there may be times when you need one or more of them. In many cases they can be of great help, but too often they have trouble seeing beyond their standard practice. And in an unfortunate and ironic way, standard practice may be the greatest contributing factor in today's chronic neck and back pain epidemic. The key is to find the right professional, for the right reason, at the right time. In chapter 7, I'll show you what to look for and, just as importantly, what to look out for.

RED FLAGS

Before you go any further, there is some vital information you must be aware of. On very rare occasions, neck or lower back pain can be a sign of a serious underlying medical condition. In these instances, the pain is usually preceded by identifiable symptoms or events that will alert you to the possibility of a serious medical problem. These warning signs or symptoms are red flags, and you should know what they are right from the start.

- significant recent trauma

- a history of osteoporosis

- a history of cancer

- a history of diabetes

- a history of kidney complications

- pain that is worse at night or when you're lying down

- unexplained fevers

- unexplained weight loss or gain

- bowel or bladder complications

If any of these red flags apply to you, I implore you to seek a qualified medical opinion before reading any further. Fortunately, less than 2 percent of neck and back pain complaints are attributable to dangerous medical conditions, and if you don't have any of the above signs, you need not be overly concerned about a serious underlying cause. Keep in mind, however, that this book is a supplement to good medical care and common sense; it is not a substitute for them. If you think you need to see a doctor, then make an appointment today.

USING THIS BOOK

The recommendations and overall experience of this book will not be the same for each person, and at times the road to recovery may seem long and arduous. Therefore, don't hesitate to read the chapters out of order. If you feel you need some motivation or reassurance, jump to chapter 8. If it's additional information about MRIs you want, go straight to chapter 5. Some ideas in this book will seem so simple and reasonable, you'll be surprised you didn't think of them yourself. Other information will be so provocative that it can change the way you think about neck and lower back pain forever.

The book has been laid out to take you through a step-by-step approach starting right at the beginning: understanding a healthy back. Old myths will be debunked, and new concepts will be advanced. You'll begin to understand how cultural influences have played a large part in transforming your acute pain into a chronic condition. You'll learn where pain comes from, what it means, and how to control and stop it. You'll be introduced to therapies, exercises, massage, and stretching, and you'll be guided through the medical and alternative approaches. In a straightforward, realistic, and practical manner, the motivation and reassurance you'll need to successfully make dramatic changes are also provided. None of this should upset your lifestyle, and you won't have to sit in a sunflower pose reciting mantras unless that's what you prefer to do.

When treating patients, I always try to keep an open ear and an open mind. If asked, patients usually aren't shy about telling me what works, and they're even less shy about telling me what doesn't. That simple but vital interaction has given me a wealth of knowledge and understanding, and now it's time for me to share that information with you. Twenty-five years of practice, thousands of patients and examinations, and hundreds of real cases have helped me formulate the core premise of this book: neck and back pain are curable.

Most of my therapy recommendations have come from patients' successes. Treatment seminars try to sell doctors specific treatments, and product salespeople have to try to sell the latest and greatest therapy, but patients call it exactly how they see it. If they've been helped, they'll tell you, and if they haven't, they'll tell it to you even louder. There are no magic bullets, miracle pills, or super high-tech solutions. You're going to have to take a good hard look at how you got into this predicament and then develop a plan to get yourself out. This book will throw you the rope, but it is your responsibility to grab on and pull like crazy. If you hold on tightly, you may be able to pull yourself right out of the downward spiral of neck and lower back pain.

THERE IS HOPE

The one idea every patient, regardless of their ailment, must sooner or later embrace is a belief that their problem can be helped. That hope is what motivates you to call a doctor, take your medicine, or buy this book. Unfortunately, too many chronic neck and back pain patients have given up hope. Today's culture has reinforced the notion that people with neck and back pain should learn to live with their problem. The expectation is for you to mask your symptoms if they get too bad, alter your life by adjusting to limitations, and complain quietly because no one is really listening anyway. Under these circumstances, how could you ever motivate or commit yourself to fighting for or finding permanent relief?

Before writing this book, I searched other resources to explore what was available. Not surprisingly, I found hundreds of back pain relief books, Web sites, and devices to choose from, all of which seemed to be lacking two key components. First, and most importantly, they completely miss the passion behind what it means to be a patient in need. The human spirit is discounted, and patients are reduced to nothing more than flesh and bones or a bundle of nerves. Sure, these resources offer techniques and procedures that can be helpful in reducing pain, but they fall far short of touching the heart of a patient in pain. In his writings, Henry David Thoreau eloquently penned the sentiments that many people with neck and back pain are feeling today: "I look over the report of the doings of a scientific association and am surprised that there is so little life to report; I am put off with a parcel of dry technical terms. Anything living is easily and naturally expressed in popular language. I cannot help suspecting that the life of these learned professors has been almost as inhuman and wooden as a rain gauge or self-registering magnetic machine. They communicate no fact which rises to the temperature of blood heat."

What I have tried to capture in this book are the facts that rise to the temperature of blood heat and the information that will stir your dreams into goals. You are more than flesh and bones, and much more than a bundle of nerves. You have the capacity to achieve great things, to overcome great obstacles, to dream great dreams, and to realize great goals. And while the physical and psychological factors that combine to produce chronic neck and back pain can be complex and intricate, you have all the necessary tools to successfully win this battle.

The second key component missing from other resources is the specific advice that turns general information into individualized procedures. They all tend to be vague, and none are dramatically better than any of the others. Many make recommendations that force you to keep pecking away at the problem. Don't you really want to just find it, fix it, and leave it alone?

If this book can open your eyes to reveal the magnificence of your body, and open your mind to change your perception of the problem, then your condition will also change. I hope you will find enough insight into the awesome wonder of your spine so you can start believing in your body's ability to control and heal itself. If you can accomplish that, then you can certainly benefit from the physical techniques in this book. Regardless of what you believe about miracles of faith, there are daily mortal miracles that result from the combination of effort and understanding. It is time to begin realizing that one of those miracles may be just around the corner for you. Although freeing yourself from chronic pain may take a huge effort, it is a goal that is physically, medically, and personally attainable.

CHAPTER 1

The Miraculous
Healthy Spine

Your spine—including all of its muscles, bones, joints, discs, and nerves—is one of the greatest structural engineering marvels of all time. This chapter will give you a basic understanding of how your spine is designed and how it works under healthy conditions. More importantly, it will also give you great respect and appreciation for the spine's amazing strength. Hard and true biological facts will replace unfounded fears and worries. Because your perceptions always affect your outcome, a basic understanding of the healthy spine is important to your recovery. With this new knowledge and appreciation in place, the road to being pain free will become much clearer. I'll start with the spinal bones and work outward, discussing the joints, ligaments, discs, muscles, and tendons. By the end of the chapter, you will realize that your back is more than just a mixed-up bundle of bothersome pain. Your spine is the miraculous backbone of your life.

THE SPINAL BONES

The bones of your back are the anchor, the base, and the living structural foundation of your entire body. Your back is composed of twenty-four individual bones called *vertebrae* that are stacked one on top of the other to make up your backbone or *spinal column.* The entire column sits on the *sacrum,* a large triangular bone that connects the spine to the hips. The top seven vertebrae in the neck are called the *cervical spine.* The next twelve segments make up the *mid back* or *thoracic spine,* and the bottom five bones in the lower back are called the *lumbar spine.* Each bone is unique in its size and shape, but they all have several things in common.

Every bone in your body is composed primarily of calcium compounds arranged into two distinct patterns. The outer bone wall, the *cortical bone,* is a very dense stonelike structure. This area is so jam-packed with dense calcium that it appears white on X-rays because low-dose diagnostic radiation cannot pass through it. The cortical bone is the bedrock of the spine. The inner bone, or *cancellous,* is arranged in a less dense honeycomb pattern that greatly reduces the overall weight of the bone and allows it to evenly distribute heavy loads to the thicker outer walls. You can think of the outer bone as granite and the inner bone as a lightweight porous rock or pumice. In contrast to the concretelike outer bone, the inner bone has a very rich blood supply and acts as a reservoir and factory for new red blood cells.

Together, these two patterns of bone create a human tissue that is pound for pound stronger than steel, yet light enough to allow you to stand erect, twist, turn, bend, and jump. These amazing structures are the anchors for your muscles and the primary support for your frame. Bone can also act like living cement. It will increase its thickness or

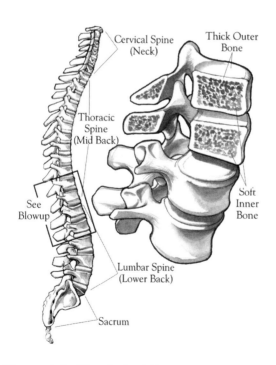

Figure 1.1: The Spinal Bones

density in areas of high structural stress, and it can replace or mend itself when fractured. Most people don't think of bone as being an adaptive tissue, but in response to weight-bearing influences it will mold itself to stabilize the spine.

Because bone is such a strong and stable structure with a limited nerve supply, it is rarely the site or origin of pain. In fact, in the absence of an uncommon disease or severe direct physical trauma, it is highly unlikely that your neck or lower back pain is coming from your bones at all. The primary function of your miraculous spine is to act as your central support, keep you upright, and protect your spinal cord. The bones are the rocks, the steel, the cement, and the foundation of your spine, and they take care of you with amazing strength and adaptability.

THE SPINAL JOINTS

Located in the rear and slightly to the sides of each vertebra, there are two top and two bottom hinges that connect the bone above and the bone below. These connections are called *spinal joints* or *articulations*. Just like any other joint in your body, spinal joints separate bones and at the same time allow them to move in very specific ranges of motion. Each joint is a uniquely shaped engineering marvel that acts as a frictionless hinge allowing for only a fraction of the motion in your spine. There are over seventy-five joints in the spine, and together they allow the entire structure to range more than 180 degrees, in any combination of up-and-down or side-to-side movements. The joint surfaces are a very hard, smooth, highly polished,

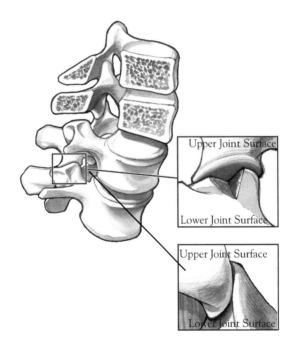

Figure 1.2: The Spinal Joints

slippery type of connective tissue called *articular cartilage*. The surfaces are separated by a thin layer of cushioning fluid, and the entire joint is held together by an extremely strong outer elastic capsule and connective wrapping called *ligaments*. The joints not only allow you to move, they also transfer weight and loads from one vertebra to the next without the bones ever touching each other.

Spinal joints are a lot like the highly polished steel shaft and casings of the hydraulic lifts you see on construction equipment. Because the bones are separated by lubricating fluid, the joints can transfer tremendous weight and pressure and still move with minimal effort. And while hydraulic lifts can move in only one direction, your joints provide movement and variability in many directions. Your spinal joints are much more than hinges. They are the strongest, most sophisticated, self-regulating, self-adjusting, and self-lubricating movement device ever designed by man or nature.

The joints are also very rich in tiny sensory nerve fibers that detect their exact position and recognize pressure. These nerves are in constant communication, creating an endless feedback loop to regulate all the joints' functions. Should a problem arise in any of the joints, the sensory nerves immediately detect the problem and coordinate that information so adjustments and corrections can be made. When all the structures, tissues, and nerves of a joint are working properly, the joint remains pain free. However, as you will see in chapter 4, if any of the joint's three main functions (holding the spine together, transferring loads, and allowing movement) becomes impaired, the nerves within the joint can become a primary source or transmitter of joint-related neck and lower back pain.

THE SPINAL LIGAMENTS

The outermost connective tissues that encase the joints and attach the bones to each other are called *spinal ligaments*. They are made up of parallel bundles of strong fibers of *collagen* (a protein-based connective tissue) that have a tremendous ability to resist pulling or stretching tensions. The ligaments also have a minimal elastic capacity, which permits limited movement. Ligaments are the steel straps that hold the bones in place. They are extensive throughout your spine, running from the base of your skull to the tip of your lower back. There are long ligaments running down the entire front and back of your

spine, there are abundant ligaments inside your spinal column, and there are also
several ligaments that fasten
each vertebra to the one
above and the one below. As
if that were not enough, there
are ligaments wrapped around
each joint, and there are more
ligaments wrapped around
each disc. There is almost no
surface of the spinal column
that does not have a ligament
attached to it.

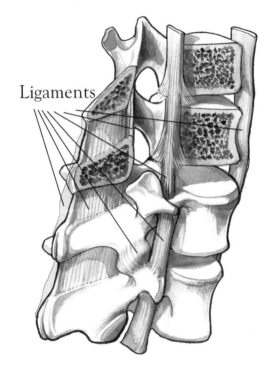

   Because the pulling
forces that ligaments must
resist are extreme enough to
damage softer blood vessels
and nerves, ligaments do not
have an extensive blood or

Figure 1.3: The Spinal Ligaments

nerve supply. Consequently, just like bone, in the absence of severe trauma,
ligaments are an unlikely source of neck and lower back pain. If they do
become injured, their limited blood and nerve supply results in a longer
recovery and healing period.

THE DISCS

Your spine is held together by more than joints and ligaments. Each bone is
also attached to and at the same time separated from the one above and below
by an intervertebral disc. The *discs* are cylindrical structures made up of a
thick, multilayered outer ring called the *annulus fibrosis* and an inner cushioning jellylike substance called the *nucleus pulposus*. The outer ring has between
ninety and a hundred layers, each composed of diagonally oriented collagen
fibers arranged in alternating angles from the adjacent layer. These layers give
the ring great strength and holding capacity, with a flexibility that allows you
to bend and turn.

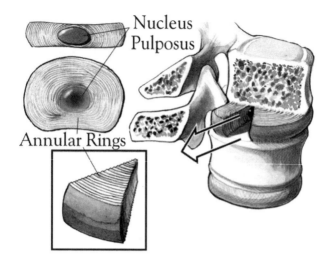

Nucleus Pulposus

Annular Rings

Figure 1.4: A Disc

The outer rings of an intervertebral disc can be compared to the tread wall of a radial tire. The layers of steel belts allow a seemingly insubstantial rubber ring filled only with air to float the weight of a two- or three-ton vehicle traveling at high speeds over bumps and around turns. An intervertebral disc works much like a tire, although turned on its side. Your discs support the weight of your body while allowing the bones to virtually float upon each other. The outer rings of the disc act like the tread wall, and the nucleus resembles the inner tube filled with air. The entire disc functions as both radial tire and shock absorber, allowing movement in all directions while providing the strength to keep you erect. The outer layers of each disc firmly attach to the outer portions of the bones and effectively hold your spine together.

The inner jellylike substance (the nucleus pulposus) acts just like the cushioning fluid in a shock absorber. In response to your position or load, it moves around within the disc to distribute both weight and force. By your twenties and thirties the nucleus begins to lose some of its water content, and as a natural consequence of aging it may actually dry up altogether later in life. The outer ring (the annulus fibrosis) has tiny nerve fibers similar to those found in joints, and these nerves can be a source of pain if the rings become disrupted or distended. And while the nucleus itself has no pain or nerve receptors, in some cases it may push through the outer ring, causing the dreaded *herniated, ruptured,* or *slipped* disc. The significance of this will be discussed in greater detail in chapter 5, but for now, keep in mind that these herniated or slipped discs are very common even in healthy, pain-free people and become the major source of irritation in only a small percentage of neck and back pain sufferers.

THE SPINAL NERVES

It's easiest to understand the nerves of the spine by dividing them into three separate groups: the spinal cord, the spinal nerve roots, and the peripheral nerve system.

The Spinal Cord

The largest group of nerves found inside the spinal column is the *spinal cord.* The spinal cord is an extension of brain tissue; along with the brain, it makes up the *central nervous system* (CNS). These nerves are the controlling core of your existence, and they are therefore encased in bone, surrounded by thick and strong ligaments, floated in their own spinal fluid, and given their own blood barrier to protect them against most of what circulates throughout the rest of your body. Although the brain and spinal cord are responsible for transmitting and registering pain, unless there is severe trauma or a rare neurological disease, the CNS is almost never directly responsible for producing neck and lower back pain.

The Spinal Nerve Roots

The next group of nerves, the *spinal nerve roots*, come directly off the spinal cord in right and left pairs of two. There are thirty-one pairs that exit the spinal column between each set of vertebrae and then travel to the rest of your body. Because nerve roots are so important for the transfer of information to and from the spinal cord, they are also housed primarily within the spinal column. They represent the transition between

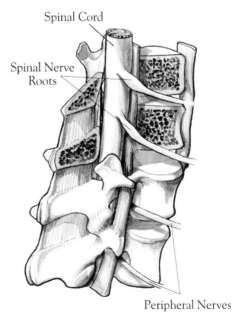

Figure 1.5: The Spinal Cord, Spinal Nerve Roots, and Peripheral Nerves

the spinal cord and your outer nerves, and they occupy the spaces between each vertebra, from which they ultimately exit. Because this is also the joint space created by a disc and two vertebrae, on rare occasions nerve roots can become impinged by herniated discs or excessive bone growth. These conditions are very painful, but direct nerve root impingement occurs in less than 5 percent of neck and back pain patients.

The Peripheral Nerve System

The last group of nerves is the *peripheral nerve system*. These nerves extend in a vast and intricate web beyond the spinal cord and nerve roots to the rest of your body. Peripheral nerves are found in every muscle, joint, tissue, and organ. These nerves are responsible for monitoring and adjusting the function of all other tissues, including those that surround your spine. Inside each joint and every muscle, there are thousands of highly specialized nerve endings that control everything from blood flow to positioning and movement. When there is a problem within any joint or muscle, it is the job of the peripheral nerves to act as the primary transmission mechanism of pain. Peripheral nerves are therefore closely associated with the sensation of pain, but they are seldom the cause of the pain. Think of peripheral nerves as messengers that alert you to existing problems.

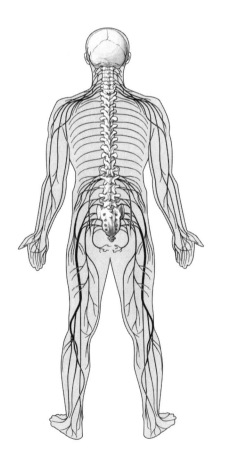

Figure 1.6: The Peripheral Nerves

THE SPINAL MUSCLES AND TENDONS

Surrounding the joints and connecting to each bone in several places are the spinal muscles and tendons. While the bones act as the frame and the joints act as the hinges, the muscles and tendons do the work that produces all the movement.

The Spinal Muscles

When muscles contract or shorten in length, bones move closer together, and when muscles relax and increase their length, bones move far-ther apart. The *spinal muscles* are made up of long banded cells that are grouped into what look like tiny threads. These threads are grouped into larger fibers, which become grouped into bundles. Finally, the bundles are woven together into individual muscles. The arrangement is similar to that of a heavy rope. The smallest fibers are intertwined to make threads, the threads are then laced together to make strings, the strings get wrapped into cords, and the cords are woven into ropes. Your muscles are structured in the same way.

Unlike rope, your muscles can stretch, contract, or hold their size and shape with great strength. When small groups of muscle cells con-tract, they cause the muscle fibers to contract. This causes the bundle to contract, and when many bundles contract

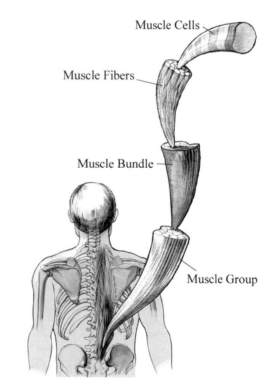

Figure 1.7: The Structure of Spinal Muscles

simultaneously, the entire muscle will shorten. All this occurs under the very specific control of tiny sensory and motor nerves within the muscle fibers and bundles. The nerves and sensors found in muscles are similar to those found in the joints. They are responsible for movement and positioning of your muscles, and are constantly telling the muscle exactly what size, shape, and strength is needed at any given moment. The relationship between the cells, fibers, bundles, and nerves is extremely intricate. The capability it gives you to fine-tune your movements is unsurpassed by any machine. Twisting, turning, lifting, bending, walking, writing, and talking are all made possible by the very fine and coordinated movements of your muscular system.

Muscles, just like bones, have the ability to adapt to external forces, and when placed under high demand, they generate great strength and power and maintain durability. To accomplish this feat, muscles can change their shape, size, and consistency. You can see these muscular changes in the sculpted physiques of athletes and bodybuilders. As they place greater demand on the muscles, the size and shape of the muscle changes in response to the demand load. And although muscle changes aren't outwardly noticeable in most people, your muscles are constantly altering their size, shape, and consistency in response to your daily activities too. Movement helps muscles maintain their elasticity, and the lack of movement causes muscles to develop some rigidity. From their very smallest component to their largest bulky mass, muscles work in unison to expand and contract. As muscle fibers change their size and shape, they glide over the surrounding fibers. The result is a living woven fabric capable of changing its size, shape, and strength depending on the demands of the moment.

Because muscles are constantly changing and adapting to produce the living equivalent of rubberized steel, they need a tremendous network of nerves to regulate their responses and a bountiful blood supply to deliver oxygen and nutrients. The intricate ingenuity of your muscles, nerves, and blood supply will be explained in greater detail in chapter 4 when I discuss the causes and treatments of muscle-related neck and lower back pain.

The Spinal Tendons

Muscles are attached to bones by fibrous bands of semielastic collagen called *tendons*. The best example of this is the Achilles tendon, which attaches the calf muscles of your lower leg to your foot. When your calf muscles contract, they pull on the tendon, which in turn moves the foot. The same is true for your spine. When your back muscles contract, they pull on tendons, which then move your spine. Like ligaments, tendons are subjected to severe pulling forces, so they too lack an extensive blood and nerve supply and must get most of their oxygen and nutrients from the surrounding tissues. Tendons have no internal or individual controls and are strictly at the pulling whim of the muscles they attach to.

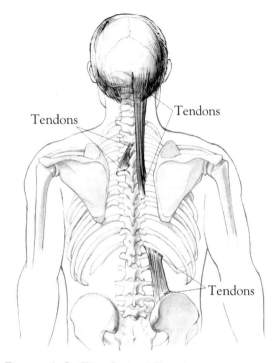

Figure 1.8: The Spinal Tendons

Tendons, just like ligaments, play a supporting role in spinal structures. Even when you are still, tendons are constantly being pulled in different directions at the same time to create a dynamic balance that keeps you upright. Without your Achilles tendon, you could not walk, and without your spinal tendons, you could not stand erect or move your spine.

Think Back

Too often, people with neck and back pain believe that their spine is nature's weak link. The models you see in a doctor's office can leave you with the impression that your back is nothing more than a string of bones limply dangling from the metal hook on a distant wall. Those inanimate models pale in comparison to the beauty and majesty of the living and dynamic human spine. Your spine is a miraculous growing, adapting structure designed to be pain free. All the tissues of your back are alive and intelligent, and they collaborate to produce a crowning element of human evolution: the ability to walk and remain upright. All the systems of your back are synchronized to create one amazing structure, the mechanical and physical design of which has never been surpassed. The key is adaptability for the good of the whole, and now you will learn how to put that adaptability to work for the good of your back.

CHAPTER 2

Myths and Misconceptions About Back Pain

Of all the medical conditions people endure, none are more confused or compounded by myths and misconceptions than uncomplicated lower back pain. As you will see in this chapter, many people attribute their pain to causes that are nothing more than myths. None of these myths are supported by reliable data, and they serve only to convince people that the pain is bewildering to diagnose and even more difficult to treat. Lower back pain is a very real phenomenon with very real physiological effects. It is difficult enough to live with pain when you are well informed and know the facts. But when your reasoning and perceptions are based on inaccurate information, it's almost impossible to zero in on a sound treatment program.

WHY MYTHS MATTER

By removing some long-held misconceptions, you can start opening up to factual and reliable information. Without a solid basis for making decisions, you are likely to remain on the chronic pain merry-go-round, spinning into more and more pain and frustration. If two patients come to a doctor's office with the exact same symptoms for the exact same problem, and one believes the condition is common and very treatable while the other believes the condition is complicated and not easily treated, the patients will likely have completely different experiences and outcomes.

This does not imply that all health problems are psychological. Rather, it suggests that the information and perceptions you have will determine how you go about resolving the problem. The better-informed patient, the one who is not thrown off track by myths or misconceptions, is in a stronger position to have a better outcome.

EIGHT MYTHS ABOUT BACK PAIN

There are other intangible variables—such as a person's emotional makeup, life views, coping strategies, and satisfaction values—that will also affect the outcome, and the importance of those issues are discussed in chapter 3. But for now, let's start clearing the way to a healthier back by removing the most common and harmful myths and misconceptions.

"I Have a Bad Back"

The first and often the worst misconception people subject themselves to is the negative and sometimes self-fulfilling statement "I have a bad back." Well, here's an important piece of information: You do not have a bad back. What you have is a wonderfully engineered, magnificently designed, and miraculously crafted human back that is unfortunately causing you pain. The myth is that because there is pain, something is significantly wrong, and consequently your back must be bad.

The truth is that regardless of where the pain is coming from, it didn't start because your back is "bad." Your back does not have a mind of its own to choose the way it will work. The spine and surrounding muscles don't choose to be good or bad, and just like every other organ in your body, they strive to perform for the good of the whole. The spinal bones and muscles are almost never the primary site of serious or life-threatening disease, and they rarely complain until neglect catches up to them when you're in your thirties or forties. Your back is a strong, flexible column allowing movement in all directions with strength and endurance well beyond what is adequate to support several times your weight. It is a shock absorber, an anchor for your limbs, and a protector of the central nervous system. It does all of this regardless of how you treat it and whether or not you pay attention to it.

Very often, the language people use to describe something is a good indicator of how they actually feel about what they are describing. Other times, the words themselves evoke feelings toward what is being described. I point this out because if you see your back as being "bad," you may treat it as if it actually were bad. What associations do you commonly make when you think about your back? "It brings up the rear." Or "It is always behind me." Or "If I can't see it, it can't bother me." Is it where you place your burdens, as in "Get off my back"? Do you think the only reason you have a back at all is to support your front? When was the last time you were at a beach and heard someone say, "Great set of traps," or "Get a load of those great-looking lats"? Is it any wonder people think of their backs as bad when everything connected with the word "back" has a less-than-front connotation?

It's about time you gave your back and spine the respect they deserve. You should herald their strengths and not presume their weakness. Stand up for your back, because it will do everything it can to stand up for you. As with a bad car or a bad boat, you may want to do anything you can to avoid the problem. But if you value your back, if you think of it as something you plan to keep around for the rest of your life, you'll look upon it and treat it with a bit more appreciation. A new attitude alone will not relieve your pain, but it will renew your commitment to treat your back in a way that may not cause you as much pain. Stop thinking of your back as being bad, and start seeing it and treating it as the only back you will ever have.

"My Back Is Out"

The next most common myth and misconception is that your back can "go out." The fact is that backs don't go out, go in, or go anywhere unless you go with them. The structure of the spine allows for a tremendous combined range of motion and flexibility. The individual spinal joints, however, each allow for only a fraction of that movement, and they are very stable structures by themselves. They are not fragile connections waiting for a wrong movement or a sneeze to send them flying out of alignment or position. In a spine where spasm and loss of movement have already occurred, the conditions are ripe for a sudden twist or a sneeze to cause significant pain. The pain may indicate you strained or sprained something in your back, but it doesn't mean your back went out of joint or position. In fact, the bones haven't moved anywhere. The amount of force required to push a spinal bone or healthy disc out of position is more likely to cause a fracture before it would cause your back to go out. This may seem like an overstatement, but for all intents and purposes, if you weren't hit by a truck, your back hasn't gone out of position.

"My back went out" is a perilous misconception because it leads you to believe that if the pain is gone, your back is "in." At that point, you are likely to ignore your back until it "goes out" again. This can foster a recurring pattern that leads to a chronic condition with more frequent episodes of longer-lasting pain. Sooner or later, you find yourself asking a very unenviable question: "Is my back in or is my back out?" Remember, backs don't go out. "Why does it seem to go out?" or "What was that popping noise?" and "What can I do to keep it from going out?" will all be addressed later. For now, let go of the misconception that your back goes out. Cars can go out of alignment, and chronic shoulder or knee dislocations can occur, but chronic back dislocations do not happen.

"My Back Hurts Because of Weak Stomach Muscles"

The idea that lower back pain comes from weak abdominal muscles is probably one of the longest running and most widely held myths among patients and many therapists, yet the basis for it remains unproven. The myth itself is illogical. It may have started from a notion that by increasing the strength of your stomach muscles, you can increase pressure in the abdomen and thereby increase support for the spine. Sorry, but you cannot. Your stomach muscles function to support the contents of your abdomen, not your back. The good news is that weak abdominal muscles have never had, and will never have, anything to do with lower back pain. Strong abs are no guarantee of a pain-free back, and weak abs are no predictor of a painful back.

Proponents of this myth would argue that millions of lower back pain patients have benefited from abdominal strengthening exercises. And while they'd be right that millions of patients have benefited, they'd be wrong about attributing those benefits to stronger stomach muscles. The beneficial effect of general exercise on lower back pain is almost universal and is extremely well documented. But no single exercise has ever been shown to be more advantageous than any other, and that includes exercises that strengthen your stomach muscles. So if you're afraid you have to do thousands of sit-ups to cure your lower back, relax. You don't. It is a myth and misconception that weak stomach muscles are a cause of lower back pain. They are not.

"It Must Be My Weight"

The next myth goes something like this: "If I could just drop a few pounds, I'm sure my back would feel a lot better." Well, you may be right, but again, not for the right reason. Just as weak stomach muscles are not a risk factor for lower back pain, neither is weight. This may come as a great surprise, but the incidence of lower back pain in the obese population is virtually the same as in the general population. The slightly greater rate of lower back pain seen with obesity is explained by *comorbidity,* the combination of a number of different illnesses or symptom complexes at one time. If obesity were a direct cause or precursor to lower back pain, we would expect to find a much higher incidence of lower back pain in that population, and we don't find that at all.

Structurally, your spine is designed to carry and support many times your body weight. Of course there must be limits, and I'm not suggesting you push yourself to find out what those limits are, but the extra body weight most people carry never approaches an amount of weight your spine could not tolerate. (While obesity may not be a major risk factor for lower back pain, it is a risk factor for other serious conditions, including high blood pressure, heart disease, diabetes, and certain forms of cancer. Keeping your weight within a healthy range is a powerful way to help prevent these medical problems.)

For weight loss, diet and exercise together have been shown to produce the best results. The reason the "drop a few pounds" myth became popular is twofold. First, because most people trying to lose weight usually incorporate an exercise program into their routine, they not only lose weight but also enjoy the other benefits that exercise in general will produce. And it is the general effect of exercise that resolves lower back pain; the diet and weight loss contribute little if anything to the favorable outcome.

Secondly, and maybe just as importantly, there are the psychological benefits of feeling better about yourself when you achieve a goal and shed a few pounds. Most people who choose to diet do so because they aren't feeling too great about their appearance, their health, or both. Once they begin to lose some weight, they start feeling better about the initial reason for losing weight, and soon they begin feeling better about secondary issues as well—including things like back pain. We all know that someone who has just lost a few pounds usually has a lighter outlook about the world in general. It is almost as though once they started feeling better physically, they started feeling better psychologically. Or it may have been the other way around; once they started feeling better psychologically, they started feeling better physically. This doesn't mean that the pain was in their head. I'm not suggest-ing that at all. However, as you'll see in chapter 3, their lighter psychological weight may have been more beneficial in reducing lower back pain than their actual reduction in pounds.

If you suffer from lower back pain and also struggle with weight issues, don't despair that until you lose the weight your back pain will continue. The two issues are entirely separate. Though I'm not recommending it, you can be pain free and overweight at the same time. If you mistakenly convince your-self that back pain and weight are inevitably linked, you may be setting your-self up for a difficult battle on both fronts. Work on conquering each as a separate entity. As you begin to make progress in one area, you'll gain the strength and determination to continue your battle in the other area as well. If you link the two together, you run the risk of not succeeding in one area and then giving up on both. Being overweight and having back pain are two separate issues, and you'll be more successful if you treat them that way.

"I Wasn't Meant to Walk on Two Legs"

This myth implies that your pain is a consequence of not being evolved enough to walk upright on two legs without pain. The theory is that because humans developed from lower primates that walk on all fours, the spine is not fully equipped for erect posture and bipedal walking. Many people believe the spine is a weak evolutionary link, the last drawback before humans fully mature into evolution's ultimate design. Look at us now: We went to all the trouble of shortening our arms, retracting our tails, shedding our fur, and then walking upright, and what is the price we pay for all that evolutionary advancement? Sciatica, thank you very much. Just make sure your pain-free friends don't find out you're plagued by one of nature's weakest links. They may stop visiting your cave and accompanying you on those big game hunting expeditions.

As you saw in chapter 1, your spine is a structural masterpiece befitting the million years of evolution over which it has developed. And although additional evolutionary improvements will occur as life and time progress, there is nothing in the current understanding of dynamic biomechanics or human evolution that gives any credence to the idea that we haven't evolved enough to be able to walk on two legs and remain upright without having pain.

In terms of what we weren't designed to do, it is possible that standing in one place and lifting machinery onto a conveyer belt for eight hours or sitting staring straight ahead at a computer screen all day are slightly beyond nature's present design specifications. However, standing upright and walking on two legs is exactly what we have spent all our evolutionary past perfecting. Besides, from a practical perspective, how could this idea lead to effective treatment for back pain? Even if you accept the theory of evolutionary inadequacy, the only thing you can do is complain, then wait another fifty or sixty thousand years and hope for some changes. That surely isn't going to help anyone today, is it?

"It's My Parents' Fault"

The myth that back pain can "run in the family" causes a defeatist resignation. Let's take a look at some sobering statistics. An estimated 80 percent of the population will suffer at least one episode of acute back pain at some point in life (Zanni and Wick 2003). At any given time, 20 percent of the population and half of working age adults suffer lower back pain (Bartleson 2001). Neck and back pain are the second leading cause of medical office visits and the leading cause of lost work time in the United States (Agency for Health Care Policy and Research 1994). Now, is it any wonder that lower back pain runs in your family? At these levels, it runs in just about everyone's family. Neck and back pain are epidemic in our society, and nothing is being done to change that. If you were born before 1965, it would be unlikely for you not to have experienced—or known someone who has experienced—significant lower back or neck pain.

Heredity plays a huge role in your medical history, and as a part of that inheritance you display body types, features, and tendencies very similar to those of your parents. These tendencies, however, are not written in genetic stone. Just because one or both parents lived with lower back pain doesn't mean you have to live with lower back pain too. The reason life expectancy and quality of life have increased significantly in the last hundred years is that each generation has learned from and improved upon the past, and so it will be with neck and lower back pain. It's time to learn from and improve upon your past.

Besides, if neck or back pain is inherited, why do we have more back pain than our parents had? They had harder, more physically demanding lives with less creature comforts. Yet, in terms of the impact back pain has on society, we have far surpassed their pain and suffering. Perhaps there are lots of things we can find to blame on our parents, but the present state of neck and back pain in this country is not one of them. If you're looking for someone or something else to blame, good luck in your search. But, with all due respect to heredity and to your parents, it's time you got off their backs about your pain.

"It Will Just Go Away"

The myth or misconception that is most responsible for getting patients into trouble is the "I thought the pain would just go away" myth. While mild, insidious pain is often self-resolving, after five to seven days of stiffness, tightness, or spasm, tissue changes occur that start developing into chronic, recurring pain. Like an achy tooth, this mild, tolerable, and seemingly benign pain now begins to return with ever-increasing frequency and intensity. If you do nothing about it for a long enough time, you are inviting yourself into the 20 percent of the population who suffer chronic neck and back pain. Maybe the pain will just go away, but if you haven't noticed it becoming progressively better after a few days, you've waited long enough. Acute pain is much easier to treat and resolve than chronic, recurring pain. And, as you will see in chapter 8, it is now well recognized that when dealing with an acute condition, the single most important initial treatment goal is to avoid the pitfalls that lead to chronic pain. Doing nothing and thinking the pain may just go away is possibly the biggest myth or misconception that can lead to chronic pain.

"Technology Will Save Me"

The last misconception, the assumption that high tech holds high hope, may be the greatest contributor to society's neck and back pain epidemic. This myth is responsible for upward spiraling costs without producing any measurable patient benefits. In patients who have red flags for severe spinal compromise, high-tech diagnostic and therapeutic procedures are warranted and can offer miraculous benefits. But in the 95 percent of uncomplicated cases, high-tech procedures—including CAT scans, MRIs, and electro-diagnostic testing—have produced few patient benefits.

In the search to find the cause of neck and back pain, researchers have uncovered a very revealing but often overlooked fact. Most of the suspected causes, including degenerative disc disease, bulging or herniated discs, and spinal curvatures, are frequently found in people who have never had one day of neck or back pain. People come in all shapes and sizes, and so do their spines. Degenerative disc disease is found in 30 percent of the normal, pain-free population (Wiesel et al. 1984); up to 40 percent of the general population has one or more significant disc changes (Jensen et al. 1994); and left- or right-sided spinal curvatures are so common that perfectly straight spines are rarer than somewhat curved spines.

The most revealing source of important clinical information is a low-tech procedure: the fifteen-minute routine history and physical examination. Much of what any good doctor needs to accurately diagnose and treat neck and lower back pain is easily obtained through a careful history of the onset of the problem, the pain's characteristics, the patient's reflexes and sensitivity to pinprick, and a few simple pushing, pulling, or stretching tests. Unless you have severe, constant neurological symptoms that have not responded to at least four weeks of conservative therapy, there is no need to undergo dangerous, costly, and time-consuming testing. And obviously the high-tech, risky, aggressive, and invasive treatments should always be reserved for the most severe and unrelenting cases. As you will see in the next chapter, advanced diagnostic testing in the early stages of uncomplicated neck and lower back pain has not been shown to influence either the treatment protocols or the final outcome.

If you're like most people, when you go to a doctor, you like to think you're getting the latest and greatest that medicine has to offer. In the case of neck and back pain, excessive diagnostic testing can lead to excessive treatment, which leads to patient dependency and chronic pain. In fact, the leading cause of chronic pain may be well-intentioned but ineffective overtreatment of the problem. With all our high-tech equipment, you would hope to see a decline in the incidence, costs, and disability incurred by these conditions, but that has not happened. While great advances have been made in spinal surgery, for the 95 percent of patients who do not require back surgery, high tech has not yielded high hopes, and all those advances have not yielded much less pain than people had twenty years ago.

Think Back

Most of what people believe about neck or lower back pain is derived from twentieth-century myths and misconceptions. Replacing those unfounded, outdated, and irrelevant ideas with new, accurate information is the first step on the road to recovery. In this chapter, I've exposed eight major misconceptions about neck and lower back pain. The "bad back" myth is an insult to how wonderful your back really is. The "my back is out" myth couldn't be further from the truth: your back hasn't gone anywhere. The "weak stomach muscles" theory remains unproven and is responsible for a lot of unnecessary, arduous, and ineffective treatment. Attributing back pain to excess weight doesn't explain the high rate of neck or lower back pain across all weight categories. The "I wasn't meant to walk on two legs" myth is silly and just plain wrong. Your ability to stand and walk upright is the culmination of a million years of evolution. Blaming heredity creates the false sense that back pain is inevitable. Maybe your back pain will "just go away," but if you are reading this book, it probably hasn't. High tech holds high hopes for people who have spinal cord or spinal nerve compression, but for the other 95 percent of neck and back pain sufferers, twenty years of high tech has not fixed—and will not fix—the problem.

In chapter 1, you learned how wonderful, strong, dynamic, and adaptive your spine really is, and in this chapter, you learned that many common beliefs about back pain are unfounded. Together, these chapters should have given you a better appreciation and understanding of your spine, allowing the full awe of nature's engineering masterpiece to shine through. This understanding can translate into greater treatment effectiveness with better results. But before we move on to the physical causes and specific remedies for your pain, one more extremely important question must be answered: can you really change your perceptions?

CHAPTER 3

Cultural Back Pain

Our bones are as strong as lightweight steel, our muscles as functional as elastic cables, our joints as versatile as space-age hinges, and our nerves as informed as supercomputers. So why, with an abundance of the most sophisticated engineering nature has to offer, has the cost and suffering of neck and back pain steadily risen over the past three decades? Understanding the mechanisms of pain and the interactions between muscles, bones, joints, discs, and nerves doesn't fully explain why chronic neck and lower back pain have become rampant across the country. The one factor that remains poorly understood and highly controversial is the degree to which psychological or emotional states contribute to chronic pain. Is the pain in your spine, or is it in your head?

Research into this subject produces undeniable evidence that a psychological component does exist with chronic neck and back pain (Linton 2000; Pincus et al. 2002). As a matter of fact, the links between back pain and psychosocial issues are so strong that all the best predictors of chronic pain and disability are psychological factors, not clinical or diagnostic ones (Carragee et al. 2005; Jarvik et al. 2005). Neither X-rays, MRIs, nor clinical findings give a reliable forecast as to who is likely to develop chronic pain. A recent study at the Stanford University School of Medicine points to poor coping skills as a more accurate predictor of future lower back pain than MRI images of cracks in discs (Carragee et al. 2004). The volume of research connecting psychological and coping strategies to chronic neck and back pain is so compelling that this issue must be considered during the initial diagnostic workup and also as a primary treatment option (Burton et al. 2004; Soderlund and Lindberg 2003). However, this does not mean that patients are generating the pain in their head as the result of a psychological disorder. The psychological component of neck and lower back pain results more from learned cultural flaws than from an individual's psychological issues.

There are times when psychological problems can cause physical pain, and it is an unfortunate fact that there are some people for whom chronic pain serves a psychological purpose. Job dissatisfaction, financial difficulties, and family stresses have all been linked to prolonged pain and disability. And while these links have been ignored for too long in favor of purely physical explanations, they do not address the vast majority of neck and back pain sufferers who desire to function fully at home, at work, and in society. For them, chronic neck and back pain serves no purpose.

Unless we are ready to concede that a large percentage of society has deep-rooted psychological distress, we must find a better explanation for the chronic neck and back pain epidemic. Embracing an unproven theory that the pain is caused by psychological stress adds to the confusion and may even create a good deal of unnecessary psychological stress in otherwise normal people. Most cases of chronic back pain begin as normally adjusted people beset with ineffectively treated acute or developing pain. Our culture's role in transforming acute pain to chronic pain through misguided theories and ineffective treatments is the basis for this chapter.

PERSONAL EXPECTATIONS

The transition from acute pain (which lasts for a few days) to chronic pain (which persists for more than a few months) is highly dependent upon psychological factors. And just as the physical transition from acute to chronic pain can be broken down and explained step-by-step, so can the psychological transition (Buer and Linton 2002; Vlaeyen and Linton 2000). Every day, you call upon your perceptions, values, knowledge, and past experiences to interpret your health. Then, based upon those interpretations, you formulate expectations that will have a greater impact on the final outcome of your health than the physical treatments will (Kalauokalani et al. 2001).

But what if the knowledge you used or the perception you had was wrong? Wouldn't your expectations and outcomes necessarily be misguided by the erroneous information? Your personal expectations are the foundation of how you cope with your problem, and they ultimately boil down to a measure of how much pain, disability, or discomfort you think you'll have. As such, most people tend to deal with pain in one of two ways: they either minimize (underreact to) pain or catastrophize (overreact to) pain, and then act accordingly.

Minimizers. People who minimize pain usually believe the situation is manageable and expect to be better in a reasonably short time. They respond by resuming normal activities as soon as possible, and that produces a greater chance of increased movement and a faster resolution of the pain-producing cycles you will learn about in chapter 4. Consequently, if all goes well, the chance of developing chronic pain should in fact be minimized. Yet these people can develop chronic pain by resuming full activities too soon or not paying enough attention to minor flare-ups that increase in frequency or intensity. A person who minimizes pain may underestimate the original injury and fail to give the tissues time to heal properly. A poor healing pattern develops that physically produces chronic pain. A minizer's mistake of undertreating an acute situation and allowing it to become chronic is not indicative of a psychological flaw, nor does it indicate a psychosomatic basis for the chronic pain. Minimizers avoid dealing with pain and getting proper treatments, and then accept the result as a normal, chronic, livable condition.

Catastrophizers. The second group of chronic neck and back pain sufferers unintentionally overreacts to or catastrophizes pain. They often perceive their initial pain as serious enough to be "backbreaking." With their perception of the situation being somewhat catastrophic, it becomes entirely reasonable, almost logical, to project an equally dire long-term expectation to match that perception. They assume that such significant pain must indicate an equally significant injury and that significant injuries usually become chronic.

The Fear-Avoidance Response and Physical Pain

With catastrophizers' beliefs firmly established on these perceptions and expectations, two additional reasonable reactions occur. First, it is easy to become unnerved by the severity of such pain to the point of developing an unrealistic fear of further pain or injury. And second, this fear can lead a person to avoid the very movements necessary to encourage proper healing. A large percentage of chronic neck and back pain sufferers finally come to display what is now called the *fear-avoidance response.*

In the very early stages of significant pain, fear and avoidance are wise and reasonable reactions. But staying in such a protective mode too long begins a series of events that will inevitably lead to chronic pain. Instead of returning to normal daily activities as soon as possible, fear-avoidant people become sedentary and guarded. Joints become restricted, muscle rigidity leads to spasms and adhesions, and a physiological cycle that produces chronic pain becomes activated. All of this gives additional credence to the patient's dire expectations and fear of chronicity. The transition from acute to chronic pain was not the result of a psychological flaw, nor was the initial pain in the person's head. Yet perceptions and values forecast the outcome and dictated how the person responded to, treated, and coped with the condition.

Fear-avoidance is a learned behavior, and people form many of their perceptions and expectations from knowing or hearing of other people who developed chronic pain in similar situations (Ferrari, Russell, and Richter 2001). These culturally learned responses explain why so many people see their own predicament in a fearful and apprehensive light. Fear-avoidant patients tend to seek treatment from multiple medical specialists, and because physical signs aren't always apparent, a doctor's casual dismissal of their pain will only reinforce their already detrimental fear and avoidance behavior (Glenton 2003).

The two characteristics minimizers and catastrophizers of pain share are avoidance and acceptance. In order to resume their daily lives, they avoid the pain or the situations they think will aggravate it, and they ultimately accept that the pain may always be there. While many patients continue seeking cures and temporary relief wherever they can find them, most will stop the search and learn to live with pain (Croft et al. 1998). Their pain, their fearful expectations, and their avoidance form a psychological chronic pain cycle similar to the chronic physical pain cycle that will be described in chapter 4. Pain evokes fearful expectations. Fearful expectations promote avoidance. Avoidance causes additional tightness and pain in joints and muscles. Additional tightness and pain evokes more fearful expectations. The next thing you know, around and around you go. Throw some work-related, financial, or marital stress into the mix, and you have the perfect recipe for alleged psychosomatic pain.

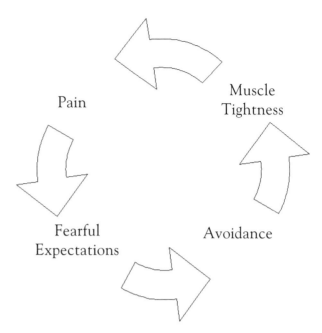

Figure 3.1: Chronic Pain Psychological Cycle

But break the cycle anywhere and it collapses like a house of cards. This doesn't mean the pain was all in your head, but by changing your expectations, you also change your fear and avoidance. You no longer confine yourself to tight and restricted postures, waiting for the next emotional or physical strain to increase the tightness to the point of pain. When you understand that pain—regardless of how severe it may be—is gone when the problem is gone, and you know that your body constantly heals itself, you can expect a bright and pain-free future.

Fear-Avoidance and Psychological Factors

Before fear and avoidance behavior was as widely accepted as it is today, some theorists believed that most chronic neck and back pain was psychosomatic, a result of the patient's mental state. Despite the lack of scientific proof, it became popular to blame chronic back pain on unresolved emotional issues, such as anger and resentment or the common stresses of money, work, and marital problems. This led to psychological treatments for chronic back pain that—amazingly enough—produced results similar to those of most other back pain therapies. Thus, over the past twenty years, psychosomatic theories and psychological treatments have become increasingly accepted and popular.

What emotional theorists did not realize was that when the cause of a patient's physical complaints was transferred to a curable psychological issue, the fear-avoidance behavior associated with physical pain was no longer necessary or appropriate, and the cycle of chronic pain was broken. Instead of an unexplained physical ailment, patients were now given a curable psychological issue which, when successfully treated, was blamed for their chronic pain. Right from the beginning, the problem was always the fear-avoidance response to pain. Seldom is the pain solely a result of psychosomatic illness. This distinction is subtle but vital, because if the psychosomatic theory is continually advanced without credible confirmation, 30 percent of the population may end up on couches blaming their parents, spouses, bosses, or friends for pain that is caused by their own fear-avoidant behavior.

The early advocates of the mind-body connection must be recognized for their breakthroughs and achievements. They uncovered much of what is now known about fear-avoidance behavior. They have changed treatment approaches so dramatically that today, a doctor who doesn't take into account a patient's fear-avoidance behavior may actually be sentencing the person to a lifetime of chronic pain. The differences between being psychologically distressed and physically fear avoidant will become clearer as you read on.

When Pain Serves a Psychological Purpose

There are some people who do have medically diagnosable psychological conditions that deserve special consideration. These are our family, friends, and neighbors for whom debilitating pain does serve a psychological purpose. The most common cause of psychologically enhanced chronic neck and back pain is job dissatisfaction. Being in so much pain that you couldn't go to work even if you wanted to may be a person's only way to safeguard their dignity while avoiding a workplace that provides nothing but disdain or discontentment. And as unimaginable or upsetting as that may seem, it is far sadder when people manifest chronic neck or back pain as a means of garnering the attention or affection they so deeply deserve. In severe cases such as these, the degree of chronic pain can be psychologically amplified to the point that it creates a devastating physical disability. These patients need compassionate, specialized treatments for their psychological conditions. They also require the utmost reassurance that with effort and dedication, they can overcome their physical pain.

CULTURAL EXPECTATIONS

Scores of studies now document the importance of gender, age, geography, nationality, economic status, and educational level in the development of chronic neck and back pain. And, as you might expect, each group has different perceptions, values, expectations, and outcomes. There are obvious factors—such as heavy labor jobs or advanced age—that account for some differences, but essentially our spines are all the same. So why are lower education, lower income, and female gender all greater risk factors for developing chronic pain (Dionne et al. 2001; Edwards, Augustson, and Fillingim 2003)? Why is a New York City cabbie more vulnerable to chronic whiplash symptoms following a rear-end accident than his Athens counterpart (Partheni et al. 2000)? After all, car accidents are car accidents regardless of where they occur, but whiplash is only whiplash if you live in certain cities. What is it about our culture that creates these differences?

Whether it's about your health, political views, or religion, cultural influences have played a vital role in everything you have learned. And, although the transition from acute to chronic pain is highly dependent upon psychological factors, those very factors are highly dependent upon cultural influences. The beginning of the transition has more to do with cultural flaws than it does with a person's maladaptive psychological perspective. If a culture teaches and reinforces maladaptive behavior, then it is not psychologically inappropriate to exhibit that behavior. Displaying the very behavior that has constantly surrounded you, even in the face of poor results, makes you an innocent casualty of society's misperceptions, not simply a person with poor coping skills. How can you be expected to know the appropriate coping skill for your condition when you have never been taught or shown those skills? If we could go back in time and wipe clean the slate of today's cultural perspectives on neck and back pain, then rewrite the script, you'd see a totally different picture.

Societal expectations, just like individual expectations, are important factors in the development of chronic pain. While whiplash is a common diagnosis in the United States, in Lithuania, where there are generally no societal expectations of complications following automobile accidents, whiplash syndrome is almost nonexistent (Obelieniene et al. 1999), and in Greece, whiplash symptoms are usually self-limiting and seldom become chronic (Ferrari, Constantoyannis, and Papadakis 2003). Though outdated cultural expectations and experiences are still dictating today's trends, they can be changed with new and better information.

But first you need to understand how the current cultural perspectives have become so deeply entrenched. There are two excellent examples of how cultural expectations about back problems have led to fear-avoidance. First, consider that years ago soft neck collars were routinely prescribed for minor neck sprains. The theory was that if the neck was injured, it should be immobilized until it healed. The rule was to avoid any further pain or injury at all costs. Patients demanded and wore their neck collars, fearing that if they didn't, they would have additional injury or increased pain. As it turns out, the exact opposite is true. For minor neck injuries, we now know that early movement is good, and the sooner you return to your normal activities, the better off you are going to be. The initial unfounded fear and the avoidance of pain led to actions (wearing collars) that increased pain and delayed healing (McKinney 1989). Imagine how fearful patients must have been when they finally took the collars off and the pain was actually worse than when they started. Who wouldn't become afraid and avoidant and expect the condition to become chronic?

The second example is the past failed approach to acute lower back pain. It wasn't long ago that bed rest and traction were the standard treatments, and if you weren't afraid of back pain before treatment, you would be after. Picture yourself lying flat on your back while your legs are pulled from your hips by a medieval-looking traction device at the end of the bed. If that's not scary enough, imagine getting out of bed one week later to find the pain is no better. What would your expectations be?

In the 1950s and '60s, almost every aspect of the treatment of neck and back pain was based upon the fear and avoidance of pain. And as it turns out, almost all of it was counterproductive. Instead of encouraging patients to resume their normal routines as soon as possible, physicians prescribed rest and restrictions. Those widespread recommendations—based strictly on the theory of avoiding pain and without any supporting scientific evidence—are the basis for today's cultural fear and avoidance behaviors. These well-intentioned but disastrous perceptions and prescriptions have made our current chronic neck and back pain epidemic the largest *iatrogenic* (doctor-induced) syndrome the world has ever seen.

Patient Responses and Perceptions

Until recently, our cultural expectations and fear-avoidance behavior typically led people with back pain to one of three experiences, each of which had its own characteristic outcome.

"BACK PAIN IS NO BIG DEAL"

The first group, the lucky ones, were given pain medication and muscle relaxers and told the problem would go away in a few days. In many cases that was exactly what happened, and the doctor and patient were both reasonably satisfied. Back pain was dismissed as nothing more than a minor nuisance, and this led to expectation number one: Most neck and lower back pain is no big deal, easily treated and just as easily dismissed. There is little need for extensive investigation or treatment, and more importantly, there is even less need for worry. Although this perception is somewhat accurate, it was eventually undermined by patient demands for newer and better treatments.

"BACK PAIN IS ALL IN YOUR HEAD"

The next group of patients weren't quite as fortunate. The limited benefits they received from treatment came only in the form of temporary relief. While the physical cause of their pain remained incorrectly diagnosed and ineffectively treated, they were subjected to ever-increasing episodes of more and more pain. Alternative therapies were not widely recognized, pain mechanisms were not fully understood, and most patients were probably seeing doctors who believed that everything could be cured with a pill or a shot. Patients and doctors searched in vain for reasonable explanations and effective remedies. Frustrated by the situation and with each other, patients began seeing doctors as unknowing and uncaring, and doctors began to see patients as hysterical hypochondriacs. Patients were left to quietly bear their pain without much hope of permanent relief, and most doctors believed that if they couldn't find or cure the physical cause, the pain must be in the patient's head. This lead to expectation number two: If neck and back pain doesn't respond to bed rest and pills, it may become a chronic condition that is not easily treated or resolved and may actually be all in the patient's head. This is the beginning of the cultural perspective that chronic neck and back pain sufferers are psychologically maladjusted.

"SEVERE BACK PAIN REQUIRES SURGERY"

The third group of patients were the least fortunate because their pain became so intolerable they eventually had to submit to surgery. Until the mid-1990s, back pain surgery was extremely unrefined, and 50 percent of patients were no better or possibly worse after treatment. The most reliable diagnostic test at the time was a CT *scan* (cross-sectional X-ray) with *myelogram* (dye injected into the spinal canal). The test had its own list of side effects that included pain, headaches, and infection. Consequently, CT myelograms were performed in only the most severe cases, and doctors saw a very large percentage of herniated discs associated with severe neck and back pain. The correct interpretation in most cases was that the herniated disc was causing the patient's pain. The error then made by some doctors and by almost all patients was an illogical assumption that *all* herniated discs cause pain. (As you will see in chapter 5, they don't.) This led to expectation number three: Severe neck and back pain is caused by herniated discs, which can only be treated with dangerous but often ineffective surgery. As far as patients were concerned, this was the scariest prospect of all. If the specter of a dangerous, painful, and ineffective surgery doesn't produce fear and avoidance in the cultural consciousness, then nothing will.

We now have three firmly implanted perspectives and expectations about back pain:

1. This kind of pain is not serious and usually goes away in a short time.

2. Neck and back pain that does not resolve in a short time is likely to become chronic and may be in the patient's head.

3. The most severe neck and lower back pain cases are caused by herniated discs that require dangerous surgical corrections.

These perceptions became so much a part of our cultural understanding that even today, if you ask any person about neck or lower back pain, you will likely get one of these responses.

New Tools and Technologies

Two other very significant influences were developing in the late 1970s and early 1980s that would eventually transform neck and back pain patients from quiet, disgruntled sufferers to voracious consumers of medical technology and services. These new services and technologies were nothing short of miraculous for the millions of patients who benefited from their best and most appropriate use, but for the rest of society, they have had the opposite effect. By further dampening expectations and barely changing outcomes, excessive diagnostic and treatment services have significantly prospered from and contributed to the fear out of which they were born.

MAGNETIC RESONANCE IMAGING

The greatest change in the diagnosis of neck and lower back pain came in the early 1980s. With the advent of *magnetic resonance imaging* (MRI), it became possible to see the bones, nerves, discs, and joints on one image without the side effects and dangers of CT scan with myelogram. Millions of patients whose condition may not have warranted a CT scan—or who were simply unwilling to undergo one—could now have an MRI to diagnose their pain once and for all. And, as you might expect, millions of eager patients with tolerable but nonresolving neck and back pain began to line up for the test. And while the technology made a quantum leap forward in a doctor's ability to safely look inside, all it really provided was a better anatomical picture, not necessarily better understanding. When MRIs revealed previously undiagnosed herniated discs, almost overnight patients' situations became intolerable. They felt an urgent need to get more medical treatment, and that is exactly what they demanded from their doctors.

ALTERNATIVE THERAPIES

Around the same time, alternative therapies were becoming more widely recognized and much more popular. Chiropractors, physical therapists, massage therapists, and acupuncturists began opening offices and colleges throughout the country. Eager to build successful practices, these professionals targeted the abundance of neck and back pain sufferers and began to apply their treatments. For the most part, alternative therapies are very helpful in alleviating day-to-day symptoms, and they give physicians another avenue to try to satisfy patients' unmet demands for more care. However, alternative practitioners did not educate patients about the consequences of fear-avoidance or teach them how to sustain long-term corrective changes. Consequently, they were unsuccessful in changing long-term outcomes. Patients came to rely on these therapies for continued relief of chronic flare-ups and even for regular maintenance. Instead of finding it, fixing it, and leaving it alone, these therapies created an entire subgroup of patients who became treatment dependent.

AN INDUSTRY IS BORN

A new but overemphasized diagnostic test (MRI), the desire to fulfill patients' needs, decades of fear-avoidance, and the mainstreaming of alternative therapies all combined to become a powerful catalyst for the dramatic and profitable growth of the neck and back pain industry. Patients are no longer relegated to quiet suffering at home; they now have the means and motivation to find new outlets through overdiagnosis and treatment dependence. The incidence and costs of neck and back pain have skyrocketed, due to advanced diagnostic testing and a plethora of *physiatrists* (doctors who specialize in physical rehabilitation), chiropractors, physical therapists, massage therapists, acupuncturists, and psychologists. As a society, we are not getting any better, and in fact the leading cause of chronic neck and back pain in the United States has become well-intentioned but inappropriately excessive testing and treatment (Livingston 1992). By their own complacency or unwillingness to address fear-avoidance, and with overzealous testing and treatment, health care professionals have become the largest contributors to today's chronic pain culture (Ehrlich 2003a; Glenton 2003).

RISK FACTORS SHOW THE CULTURAL INFLUENCE ON BACK PAIN

If you need additional evidence to illustrate the cultural impact on neck and back pain, look at the various subgroups of patients who have the same spines and the same problems but entirely different outcomes. People can be divided by how they think, into *psychosocial* groups, or by how much money they make, into *socioeconomic* groups. Merely documenting that being a woman, having less of an education, or making less money all represent increased risk factors for developing chronic pain doesn't explain the pain away; it simply emphasizes the importance of a cultural connection to these problems. Health care practitioners have a social responsibility to make sure all of their patients get the message that exercise, activity, and lifestyle changes can all have beneficial effects. The obligation to see that all patients are properly informed belongs as much to the physician as it does to the patient. So, if patients fall into a socioeconomic or psychosocial group that places them in a special risk category, it is part of the doctor's treatment obligation to see that they get the special information they need and deserve. Doctors must not blame patients for not knowing information they have never been given.

■ A Case of Cultural Back Pain

In the mid-1980s, I treated a young man I'll call Tim for neck and upper back pain that occasionally traveled into his right shoulder and arm. I applied the standard therapies, including gentle massage and manipulation, and he responded favorably. I hadn't seen him for about two years when he returned complaining of lower back pain radiating into his buttock. After an updated history and physical examination, I was quite sure this was a routine case, not unlike any of hundreds of other cases I had successfully treated in the past. This was garden-variety lower back pain without signs or symptoms of a herniated disc.

Earlier that week, a sales representative from a new local MRI facility had dropped off literature on the virtues of MRI. Having recently read several articles on the subject, I was interested to see what the new technology had to offer. Tim himself had heard about MRI, so when I suggested he have the test, he was eager to comply.

A week later I received the results, and to my surprise the MRI revealed two herniated discs in Tim's lower back. At his next visit, Tim was feeling noticeably better, and we then discussed the MRI findings. I will never forget the look on his face when I told him there were two herniated discs in his back. He became visibly upset, and the blood drained from his face. He wanted a second opinion and took the MRI to an orthopedist, who confirmed the findings and told Tim to immediately stop spinal manipulation and most of his activities. This was not the first time I had seen irrational professional fear and avoidance drive a case in exactly the wrong direction, but it was one of the most obvious.

I didn't see this patient again until four years later, when I bumped into him in a supermarket. By this time, I had seen many more uncomplicated lower back cases with herniations on MRIs that responded beautifully to conservative treatments, yet surgery still remained the treatment of choice. Tim informed me that after several months of physical therapy and then bearing the pain for two more years, he finally had surgery, which he thought had gone fairly well. And while he was no longer able to enjoy long bike rides or play golf, Tim was grateful for warm, sunny days, when the pain usually wasn't too bad.

Once Tim received his MRI results, the rest of the case was driven entirely by fear and avoidance expectations as opposed to hard facts. Based upon what he and his surgeon both expected, the case turned out just fine. To this day, however, I can't help but think that had I not sent him for the MRI, had I just treated his lower back pain as I had done for hundreds of other cases like his, and had he just expected that with one or two more treatments he'd be fine, then maybe he'd still be riding his bike and playing golf today. Fortunately, spinal surgery has become much more selective and advanced than it was twenty years ago, but to a great extent, neck and lower back pain patients still face the exact same dilemmas today.

Even with better diagnostic equipment and a wider choice of reliable conservative treatments, unfounded fear-avoidance perceptions and expectations continue to produce negative results. The lure of high-tech testing and the demand for high-tech conservative and aggressive treatment have put tremendous pressure on doctors to utilize services and technologies that have not yielded the desired results. Under the right conditions, high-tech testing and treatments are miraculous. Unfortunately, their overuse and misinterpretation have greatly contributed to today's neck and back pain epidemic.

CHANGING CULTURAL EXPECTATIONS

If the neck and back pain epidemic is going to be reversed in this country, it will occur by way of a cultural change, not a medical breakthrough. This has been true of almost all the great societal epidemics. In the past, large-scale public health and sanitation programs have turned the tide, and the same will be true for today's neck and lower back pain. As a society, we have done nothing to quell our unfounded fears and dire expectations, and there doesn't seem to be any public initiative to do so. We are still hanging on to the false hope that a new therapy or technology is just around the corner. And in an ironic twist, the answer to these widespread back problems may have been staring us in the face the entire time. There is now abundant and compelling evidence that societal expectations and patient outcomes can be positively influenced through public educational and behavioral programs (Buchbinder, Jolley, and Wyatt 2001; Indahl 2004; Mootz et al. 2000).

Each year, tens of thousands of heart disease patients are being saved by new medical technologies and treatments. And as wonderful as that is, even more dramatic—though less widely publicized—are the tens of millions of patients who as a result of educational programs are avoiding the disease in the first place. Pediatricians and ear, nose, and throat physicians have recently concluded that thirty years of prescribing patient-demanded antibiotics for childhood ear infections was unnecessary and probably counterproductive. These physicians are changing their treatment protocols and asking parents to change their expectations. Will orthopedists, physical therapists, and chiropractors begin to make similar statements about their own protocols? Public education can help alleviate and prevent chronic neck and back pain and steer patients away from counterproductive treatments. The results of such an initiative are sure to be just as spectacular for chronic neck and back pain as they have been for other diseases.

What can you do as a person with neck and back pain? How can you use the idea that your pain has a cultural component to take better care of yourself? First, appreciate the dynamic strengths, structures, and healing capacities of the human spine. Reassure yourself that back pain is usually benign. Educate yourself about the consequences of fear-avoidance. Avoid the perils of ineffective, excessive, or counterproductive treatments. Don't get caught in a cycle where you're awaiting your next episode of pain and developing a treatment dependency that reinforces your perception that you have a chronic weakness and need more and more care. Most importantly, learn the behavioral techniques in this book, including targeted massage, directed stretching, directed exercise, and self-motivation.

Think Back

The longstanding debate about whether chronic neck and back pain are real or just in the patient's head is over. For all but a small percentage of unfortunate patients, chronic neck and back pain are a constellation of very real physical factors combined with personal and cultural perceptions and expectations. The transition from acute to chronic pain is significantly influenced by the physical and psychological factors that patients have learned from their surroundings. Psychological factors are more accurate in predicting future cases of lower back pain than physical factors are. The fear-avoidant approach to treating neck and lower back pain is a primary contributor to today's epidemic of neck and back pain. It has created an entire population of pain sufferers who expect their condition to become chronic and act according to those expectations. There is now sufficient compelling research to suggest that chronic neck and back pain can be greatly reduced through public education and changes in behavior.

CHAPTER 4

Muscle Pain and Its Treatment

Ninety-five percent of neck and lower back pain patients suffer nonspecific pain that is not attributable to infections, diseases, fractures, or other serious underlying medical conditions associated with the red flags listed in the introduction. If you skipped the introduction or don't remember the red flags, go back and read them now.

Because muscles represent the greatest amount of body mass and are responsible for all movement, they are the first place to look for the cause of your neck and back pain. Muscles don't begin to hurt for no reason, so something in their structure or function has to be wrong in order for you to feel pain. In this chapter, you'll find out what causes muscular back and neck pain and how to treat it effectively.

MUSCLE STRUCTURE

Let's begin by reviewing muscle anatomy. Aside from the muscle cells, fibers, bundles, and groups discussed in chapter 1, there are two important structures found in muscle that contribute to pain: connective tissue and sensory and motor nerves.

Connective Tissue

Every muscle has an interwoven connective tissue that attaches the muscle fibers and bundles together. If you picture muscles as a large, ornate stained glass window, the fibers and bundles would be the different sized colorful glass panels. The surrounding and supporting connective tissue would be the surrounding and supporting lead in the windows. This connective tissue, which looks like steak gristle in large bundles, is composed of collagen strands that give it a tremendous ability to withstand pulling or longitudinal strains. It also has limited elasticity, which allows it to stretch while still holding the tissues together. Without the connective tissue holding the muscles together, you would lose your strength and the ability to move your bones or support your frame.

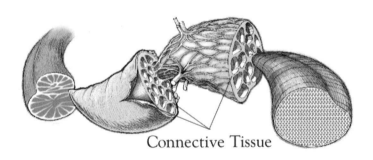

Connective Tissue

Figure 4.1: Muscle with Connective Tissues

Sensory and Motor Nerves

The second important group of structures within the muscle are the sensory and motor nerves. These nerves are responsible for positioning, movement, tone, and pain. They regulate everything from fine muscle movement that allows you to blink an eye to gross positioning of your trunk and limbs.

There are different types of nerves, and their interaction results in either a pain-free or painful neck and back.

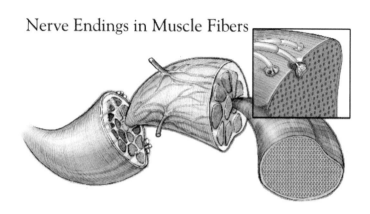

Nerve Endings in Muscle Fibers

Figure 4.2: Muscle with Nerves

Under ideal circumstances, the nerves are constantly producing and transmitting information to the spinal cord concerning movement, tone, and positioning. This information is processed in the spinal cord and brain, and responses are immediately sent back to the muscles. All of this production, transmission, processing, and retransmission sets up a continuous cycle of free-flowing information that keeps the muscles of your neck and back working properly.

This cycle has one other very important property. When normally functioning muscles and nerves are working in concert, they produce an abundance of information that inhibits pain-producing nerves from generating their impulses. The constant beneficial messages of movement and positioning allow little or no room for distressful pain signals to pass into the spinal cord or brain. Unless pain signals are turned on in overwhelming force, the body's incomparable system of prioritizing information relegates the production of most pain to nothing more than undetectable background noise.

Trauma as a Source of Muscle Pain

Trauma to muscles can come in many forms and in various degrees, from something as simple as a sneeze to an event as violent as an automobile accident. Fortunately, because your muscles are so strong, resilient, and quick to react to traumatic forces, in most cases only minimal damage can occur on a microscopic level. The largest muscle bundles generally remain intact and uninjured, while the smaller muscle fibers and the internal connective tissues are subjected to minute separations or *microtraumas*.

MICROTRAUMAS

The most common microtrauma results in an extremely localized injury only to cells, the tiny muscle fibers, and the internal connective tissues. In this type of injury, the force is enough to damage cells but not enough to damage larger bundles. The body reacts on a microscopic level, with the immune system dispatching white blood cells to clean up the damage. Some mild and undetectable swelling or loss of movement may also occur. These microtraumas are no different than the minor bumps or bruises you occasionally get on other parts of your body. The initial swelling and immobilization will temporarily inhibit movement and thereby reduce the production of normal nerve information. The reduced flow of normal nerve information allows newly stimulated pain signals to freely enter the spinal cord and brain and initiate a cycle of pain. Once the swelling has gone down and the area begins to move freely again, the pain quickly becomes blocked and diminished. These injuries usually require minimal treatment and resolve on their own in a few days without becoming chronic or debilitating.

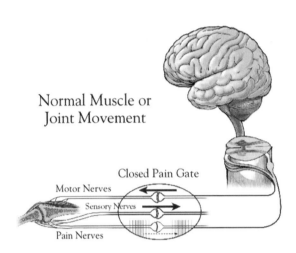

Figure 4.3: Proper Nerve Transmission Patterns

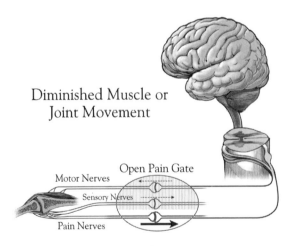

Figure 4.4: Improper Nerve Transmission Patterns

STRAINS AND SPRAINS

The second most common muscle injury or trauma is a bit more serious and comes from an actual disruption of muscle fibers or connective tissue bonds. These injuries usually happen when muscles are subjected to extreme pulling or tearing forces. *Strains* occur when the muscle fibers or connective tissue bonds become slightly separated or pulled apart by heavy lifting or forceful exertion of the muscle. *Sprains* occur when muscle or connective tissues actually become torn by the significant shearing forces of direct physical trauma. In either case, if the external forces are great enough, muscle or connective tissue bonds can be separated.

These injuries are more serious than microtraumas because the disrupted tissue bonds must be restored and reoriented in a manner that will allow free and unrestricted movement. If the bonds are restored haphazardly, weak and inflexible scar tissue will develop, and movement can be permanently lost. If that happens, chronic muscle stiffness and rigidity will occur and chronic pain can result. Under ideal circumstances, if you engage in the appropriate stretching and exercise to promote the proper reorganization of tissue patterns, these injuries can resolve in just a few weeks. However, if you don't gently stretch and exercise the muscles and the tissue heals poorly, loss of movement will persist and pain signals will continue to override normal nerve traffic.

Prolonged Positioning as a Cause of Muscle Pain

After trauma, the other leading contributor to muscular neck and lower back pain is prolonged positioning. Allowing your neck or back to remain in any one position for too long can have the same consequences as lack of movement due to trauma. The best example of prolonged positioning is sitting at a computer all day. Workers who previously had to manually file papers or physically deliver interoffice mail now perform these tasks with the click of a mouse. An unfortunate consequence of this increased office efficiency is the lost opportunity for workers to move their necks and backs. The technology itself is not the problem, but how people go about using it greatly contributes to the prolonged positioning that results in chronic neck and back pain.

Without the proper stimulation or regular movement of the muscles, irritating pain messages are able to enter the spinal cord and brain unimpeded. If this scenario is reinforced daily and continues unabated, it will create a destructive cycle of chronic pain. Instead of the proper muscle stimulation inhibiting and blocking pain, pain eventually begins to inhibit and block muscle movement. This cycle is easily perpetuated because the more pain you feel, the more you tend to restrict your activities. Instead of initiating movement that stimulates the nerves to produce normal, pain-blocking impulses, people usually allow the pain to block their movement. When you stay idle, less pain blocking occurs and more pain irritation is produced. As you lower the beneficial inputs, pain increases and the cycle becomes chronic. Finally and most devastatingly, this process will ultimately cause changes in the quality and consistency of the muscle tissues that may take months or years to reverse.

IDENTIFYING MUSCLE PAIN

Before starting any self-treatment program, it is vitally important to make sure you are treating the right problem. Therefore, the first question you need to ask is, is this muscle pain? The history of onset, the characteristics of the pain, and the location of the pain will all help answer that question. So, after you've ruled out a serious underlying medical problem or direct physical trauma such as injury from falling, being struck by an object, or being in a violent car accident, and if no red flags are present, the next step is to evaluate the history, characteristics, and location of your pain. This evaluation will provide valuable information about what may be causing the pain.

History. The primary history for the onset of muscular neck and back pain is:

- pain that began gradually or for no apparent reason

- pain that began with a mild to moderate strain

- pain that starts or gets worse after you stay in one position

Characteristics. The primary characteristics of muscular neck and back pain are:

- pain that comes and goes

- pain that is worse in the morning and gradually gets better as the day goes on

- pain that you can describe as a tightness, pulling, achiness, or soreness

- pain that with prolonged positioning causes a burning or tingling that goes away with movement

Location. The primary location of muscular pain is:

- a specific, local area the size of a fist or smaller

- a nonspecific, broad, or beltlike pattern across the central lower back

- an entire region of your neck or back (in severe cases)

Because the structures and tissues surrounding the spine are closely intertwined functionally, anatomically, and neurologically, it can be extremely difficult to identify the exact source of neck and lower back pain, and significant muscular neck or back pain may cause additional symptoms at other locations. But muscle pain is usually localized and is therefore also known as *regional pain.* Regional pain can spread outward over a wider area, with a broad gripping and tightening sensation in the muscles. On occasion, if the muscle tightening is severe enough, small nerve fibers and blood vessels can be squeezed to the point where a tingling sensation can occur in the hands or feet. This tingling is not pain, but feels more like the hand or foot is falling asleep. Regional pain may also

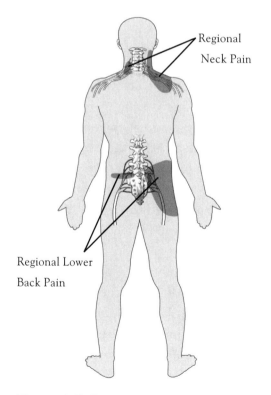

Figure 4.5: Regional Neck and Back Pain Distributions

come on suddenly and severely following trauma or injury. Regional muscular neck pain will typically run from the base of the neck down and outward, covering much of the upper shoulder blade region. Regional muscular lower back pain is most often felt from the spine outward along the crest of the hip and into the upper half of the buttock.

Unless you have severe and constant shooting, stabbing, and numbing pain in your arms or legs, your pain is most likely muscular in origin. The other sites that can produce neck and back pain (joints, discs, and nerves) will be discussed in the next chapter.

TREATING MUSCLE PAIN

By treating muscle pain promptly, you can avoid initiating a cycle of chronic pain. In this section, you'll learn the safe and effective treatments for muscular neck and back pain.

Step One: Stop the Acute Muscle Pain

Once you've determined that you probably have muscular neck or back pain, step one is simply and most importantly to stop the pain. Contrary to what many doctors, therapists, and patients believe, there will be time for finding and treating the cause of the pain later on. But in order to move forward, you first have to try to reduce the pain.

The most convenient and cost-effective initial treatment is over-the-counter pain medication. A brief course of the recommended doses of aspirin, acetaminophen (Tylenol), or ibuprofen (Advil or Motrin) can help reduce pain levels so you can resume some of your normal daily activities. Getting back to your normal routine as quickly as possible may be the most important step you can take on the road to recovery (Borchgrevink et al. 1998; Hagen, Eriksen, and Ursin 2000). Many people don't like taking medications of any kind, but short-term use of over-the-counter pain medication or prescribed *nonsteroidal anti-inflammatory drugs* (NSAIDs) can be helpful (van Tulder et al. 2000). If medication successfully reduces your pain, you will likely begin increasing your movement. The sooner that happens, the sooner you can begin a more aggressive therapy regimen. If your pain is significantly inhibiting your movement and you think you may need pain medication, take it. Avoiding medication and bearing the pain may only serve to prolong your pain and delay your recovery. The risk of developing long-term tissue damage and chronic pain is far worse than the risk of short-term side effects from pain medication.

Step Two: Treat the Acute Muscle Problems

The next step is to treat some of the immediate physical changes, including swelling, sensations of heat, and the release of loss-of-movement irritants that produce noxious pain impulses. For trauma or overexertion, two to three days of rest (minimal time in bed in addition to sleeping, and no forceful exertion) is the treatment of choice. Strained (slightly pulled) and sprained (slightly separated) tissues need time to heal and should not be taxed during the healing period. So, without being fear-avoidant, it is important to remember that insufficient rest after injury exposes you to an increased risk of further injury. However, because loss of motion can delay recovery, it's beneficial to begin gentle and comfortable movement as soon as possible. Eventually, you'll want to exercise to make sure the tissues repair themselves fully and properly, but initially, rest and gentle movement are recommended. Complete bed rest should only be considered when even minimal movement or slight weight bearing causes severe shooting or stabbing pain.

Heat and swelling are the other two physical effects of acute injury. In keeping with good common sense, if trauma gets rest and pain gets medication, then heat, swelling, and any burning pain should get ice. Make sure you protect your skin from direct contact with ice or any other cooling agents. Then apply them with caution. For neck pain, a ten-minute application is all you need. The mid back can take up to fifteen minutes, and the lower back can tolerate twenty minutes of ice. Do not go beyond these recommended times, because too much ice may actually be counterproductive. The pain-blocking effect of ice should last up to thirty minutes, and ice can be reapplied every other hour.

Starting the third day after a trauma or overexertion injury, if there is no longer any burning or swelling in the muscles, you can apply *mild,* nonpenetrating heat for no more than fifteen minutes every other hour. Prolonged heat will cause prolonged weakness, soreness, and pain and should never be used in the presence of severe sharp, shooting, or stabbing pain. As your symptoms subside, so should the treatments. The initial acute phase of an injury usually lasts just three to seven days, and these recommended treatments should not last much longer.

Step Three: Begin Targeted Deep Massage and Directed Stretching

By the fifth day after an injury, and for the next six to twelve weeks, the repair phase is under way, and the treatments begin to reflect a more proactive approach. This is the time when muscle healing and reorganization occurs, and it is essential that the repair takes place with a minimum of scarring and weakness. Excessive muscle tightness during the repair period—or in cases of chronic muscle pain—produces a pattern of disoriented fibers that reduce blood flow in the affected tissues and cause a buildup of waste products. This combination increases the likelihood that muscles will "knot up" and form areas of bound-together fibers called *adhesions,* which eventually result in painful and unrelenting spasm. Therefore, in both acute and chronic cases, during the repair and reorganization of injured muscles, the most widely indicated therapeutic approaches for alleviating muscle spasms and reducing tightness are *targeted deep massage* (Cherkin et al. 2003; Hernandez-Reif et al. 2001) and *directed stretching* (Long, Donelson, and Fung 2004; Rosenfeld, Gunnarsson, and Borenstein 2000).

Targeted deep massage and directed stretching are the dynamic duo of acute and chronic muscle pain therapies. And although many other approaches and devices are widely used to provide temporary relief, none have ever been proven to be as effective or as reliable in providing relief or influencing the final outcome. Targeted massage and directed or *directionally preferred* stretching should not be confused with general massage and general stretching. While general therapies produce limited and general results, targeted and directed therapies are site specific and yield site-specific results. Targeted deep massage and directed stretching are the therapeutic "smart bombs" of muscle-related neck and back pain. If used correctly, they will be dramatically different from anything else you have tried in the past. Joint, disc, and nerve pain will get their own site-specific therapies in the next chapter; for now, let's focus on your muscular neck and back pain.

TARGETED MASSAGE

Targeted massage is designed to disrupt the adhesions and chemical bonds that hold the muscles in spasm. When you apply targeted massage, blood, oxygen, and nutrient flow to the muscle is increased; waste products are removed; movement is restored; and nerves become stimulated to produce pain-blocking impulses. The relief may be temporary at first, but as time goes on the benefits become more substantial and longer lasting. Targeted massage begins by identifying as exactly as possible the site of the offending muscle spasm. Identifying the site makes the massage and stretching more specific and more productive. If you don't properly identify a specific site, you're using the therapies like a shotgun, blasting away at large regions hoping to hit something.

In this section, you'll learn how to target and massage muscle spasms in the neck and back. You can easily find and massage neck spasms by yourself. Targeting and massaging muscle spasms in the back is best done with help from another person, but I'll show how you can do it by yourself too.

Targeting and Massaging Muscular Neck Pain

It is easiest to identify the location of *cervical* (neck) spasm by lying flat on your back looking up at the ceiling. This relieves your neck of bearing weight, and you can search the muscles when they are more relaxed. Begin by placing your fingertips at the base of your skull, and gently press into the muscles. Then slowly run your fingers down your neck, eventually trying to cover all the areas between the base of your skull and the top of your shoulders. If very light pressure causes significant or stabbing pain in your neck or through your upper back, you are still in an acute stage, and you should not proceed. However, in most cases the light contact will feel soothing and will gently ease the tightness and pressure. This response is an indication you can proceed, and although it generally feels good, by itself the light pressure has very little if any overall benefit.

When you reach the specific offending muscle fibers, the gentle and soothing pressure will suddenly turn to a very localized sharp or ice pick–like sensation. That's your spasm. It should feel like a tiny steel wire or perhaps a small pea in the midst of softer, more pliable tissue. If you are having trouble locating the area, you can gently increase the pressure you are using. However, when working on your neck, be sure to never apply deep or heavy pressure above the shoulder level. This area contains large blood vessels and large, sensitive nerves that can be vulnerable to severe compressive forces.

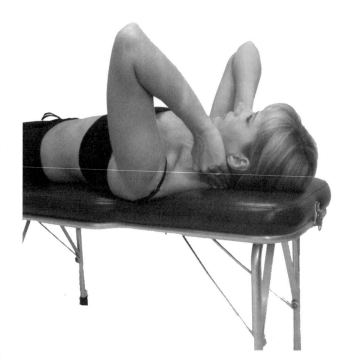

To massage neck spasm, apply firm and steady circular pressure over an area about the size of your fingertip for thirty to forty-five seconds. If you feel general

Figure 4.6: Identifying and Massaging Neck Spasm

muscle tightness in your neck, you can also safely use gentle, superficial, soothing massage over the specific site two to three times daily. There is no benefit to massaging the entire neck for long periods of time. Gentle and regular targeted massage is all that is required to reduce neck spasms.

Targeting and Massaging Muscular Back Pain

You can locate muscle spasm in your upper and lower back by lying on your stomach and having someone apply light to moderate finger pressure over the general area. Again, if this very light pressure causes significant and stabbing pain, then you are probably still in the acute phase, and you should not proceed. But just as with neck spasm, in most cases of upper or lower back pain that are at least four days past an acute injury, the light contact will usually feel soothing and produce a gentle easing of the tightness and pressure. Have the person slowly keep moving around the area until you suddenly feel a very localized sharp or stabbing sensation. That means you've found your spasm. Muscle spasms in the back will feel like a rope or perhaps a small marble embedded in softer tissue. If you're having trouble finding the spot, have your helper slowly increase the amount of pressure being applied. Don't be afraid. You won't cause additional injury or trauma.

The best place to begin your search for upper back pain is halfway between the spine and the shoulder blade on the side that feels painful. Have your helper start at the very top of your shoulder, halfway between your neck and arm, and then slowly work down between the spine and the inside edge of the shoulder blade. The upper back muscles are much thicker than the neck muscles and can tolerate deeper pressure without the risk of injury. These muscles also connect to the neck and are responsible for much of the pain, discomfort, and loss of movement associated with neck pain. Therefore, you should consider the upper back as a possible source of irritation if you have neck pain.

Once you've located the sorest or most rigid spot in the muscle, have your helper use the tips of their fingers or thumb to begin applying a localized deeper, heavier, and circular pressure to the site. You'll know this is being done properly if it hurts like all heck. And, while I have never been a proponent of the "No pain, no gain" theory, in the case of upper or lower back spasm, targeted massage really is necessary to change the consistency and tissue patterns of the muscles. Fortunately, however, there is no need to spend long periods of time doing targeted massage. One to two minutes twice daily is sufficient to begin disrupting the old adhesions and spasms and lay the foundation for a new and proper tissue pattern.

Identifying lower back spasm is done in the exact same manner. Muscles of the lower back are even thicker and denser than those of the upper back, so you may have to apply a bit more pressure. Don't be afraid of causing further injury. The best place to begin looking for lower back spasm is from the middle of the spine at waist level to about three inches outward on either side of the spine just above the crest of the hip bones. Use enough pressure so it feels somewhat soothing, but make sure it is more than just a gentle rub. If you don't use enough pressure, you may not find the spot. The spasm should feel like a rope or a marble in spongier muscle, and putting pressure on it will be painful. Even if the person applying the pressure cannot feel the rigidity or pebblelike spasm, when your helper hits the spot, you'll know it. If you are a kind and gentle soul, when the spasm is found, you'll say something like, "Ouch" or "By gosh, that's it." If you're like some of my New York patients, you may express a slightly briefer and harsher sentiment.

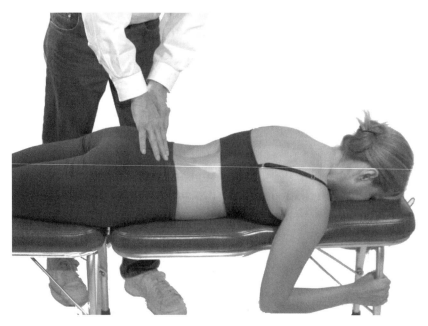

Figure 4.7: Identifying and Massaging Back Spasm

Just as with the upper back, once you've located the spasm, step two is to begin loosening its grip. Start by applying as much pressure to the spasm as you can reasonably tolerate. Have someone rub or massage the spasm with the tip of the thumb, several fingertips at one time, or the heel of the hand if necessary. As long as your helper is putting enough pressure on the right area, the exact technique isn't very important. If it is being done correctly, you will feel a sharp, almost burning pain in the spasm. Don't be afraid. Although the pressure may be painful and uncomfortable, one to two minutes twice daily will not injure you or make you worse. Pulling or straining forces cause most muscle injuries to the lower back, and the relatively light compressive forces used during targeted massage are not dangerous.

The day after your first targeted deep massage, your original painful, burning, and gripping symptoms will likely have lessened to a dull, achy pain. If the massage was very forceful, you may also feel as though you have a slight bruise or a lesser and more superficial type of pain in the area. This is a common response, and most people are more than happy to make that trade-off. Because targeted deep muscle massage is so effective in reducing severe spasm, it is only necessary to repeat this procedure three to four times weekly during the first three weeks of treatment. After that, the spasm should be significantly reduced, and so is the need for this treatment. Targeted deep muscle massage can then be applied as needed.

Targeting and Massaging Muscular Back Pain by Yourself

Targeted massage is an essential ingredient in the successful treatment of muscular neck and back pain, so even if you cannot get someone to help, you must find a way to accomplish the goal of locating and disrupting adhesions and spasm. The best technique for self-administered targeted massage to the upper and lower back is with the aid of a junior-sized basketball. Any type of tennis ball, soccer ball, or basketball can also be used, but stay away from golf balls or baseballs—they're just too hard. A tennis ball will usually slide around on a smooth wall, so you can try placing it in a doorjamb or wide corner.

You can locate the spasm by getting into a semiseated or squatting position and then placing the ball between your back and a wall. By pressing your back against the ball, you will generate the same type of pressure into the tissues that would be applied if you had someone doing it for you. Using mild to moderate pressure, slowly wiggle your body around, trying to manipulate the ball into different areas of the affected muscle. If the entire area is extremely painful or shooting pain is produced, do not continue until the procedure becomes more tolerable. Once the soothing or relaxing effect of the pressure turns to a sharp or ice pick–like pain, you have found the right spot.

With the ball firmly on the spasm, spend another one to two minutes applying heavier pressure to the site. By using a very limited up-and-down or side-to-side motion, you can produce the effect of massaging action. Do this twice daily. Some people feel more comfortable lying on their back and placing the ball between their back and the floor. A tennis ball is too small for this technique, so you'll have to use something bigger. Don't try to lie straight back onto the ball; that is much too difficult. Start by lying on your side, and then roll your back onto the ball. Also, it may help to have a chair close by so you can hold on and help stabilize yourself. If you try this technique, be sure to move slowly and under control. Remember, this is not an athletic event; it is a controlled, targeted massage.

Although this looks similar to the way people use very large, soft balls to stretch their back in gyms or physical therapy, it is actually a very different procedure. While those large balls may be good for general stretching, they do nothing to disrupt the adhesions that you are targeting with this massage technique.

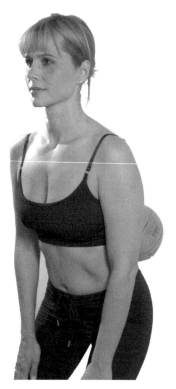

Figure 4.8: Targeting and Massaging Muscular Back Pain Using a Ball

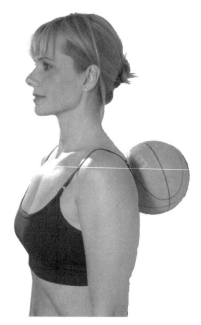

Figure 4.8B: Targeting and Massaging Muscular Back Pain Using a Ball

DIRECTED STRETCHING

Now that you've identified the muscle spasms and targeted massage has started to loosen their grip, you must keep those sites from tightening up again. Therefore, the next step is to regain motion and maintain the healthy tissue patterns you have already begun restoring. The best way to accomplish this is with a directed stretching program that will reorganize old, restrictive, and destructive tissue patterns. This unique stretching technique focuses movement at the exact site of repair. This is essential because if even a small area of spasm remains, it can eventually lead to significant tightening and renewed symptoms in larger muscle bundles. And while millions of patients temporarily benefit from nonspecific stretching of these larger muscle bundles, unless the small, specific adhesions and spasms are diminished, the tightening and discomfort will return.

The repair phase of healing is characterized by the laying down of new tissues, fibers, and collagen bonds. If there is limited movement in the muscles during this period, the fibers and bonds will be repaired in the same haphazard, twisted, knotted, and chaotic patterns that resulted in the original painful spasms and loss of motion. However, if the fibers and bonds are repaired in well-organized and layered patterns, minimal if any painful loss of movement will occur. Only regular movement in the affected muscles can ensure that the proper healing patterns will develop, and directed stretching is the best way to ensure that movement happens in the affected sites. As the normal adjacent muscle fibers and bonds continue to glide smoothly over and around each other, new cells are deposited along the gliding planes and are aligned by the gentle pulling forces. Randomly deposited cells can form adhesions, but directed stretching movements stimulate an organized pattern of repair and growth. The resulting smooth, layered, integrated pattern prevents the formation of destructive, weak, and inflexible scar tissue. In contrast, the longer stiffness and loss of movement are allowed to linger, the more extensive the scar tissue development will be. The sooner proper movement is restored, the less scar tissue is produced.

As an acute injury begins to heal or a chronic spasm begins to loosen, you naturally begin to get more movement. Gentle increases in the movement will actually relieve some of the uncomfortable stiffness and tightness by stimulating the beneficial sensory inputs that help block pain. If the injury is not too severe and gentle stretching is started soon enough, the formation of adhesions or scar tissue can be prevented. But in cases where chronic adhesions have already formed, if significant movement is not restored, then no matter what therapy you undertake, the relief will be limited and temporary. Most treatments produce only enough stimulation or movement to temporarily block pain, and few ever make enough of a correction at the specific site to achieve lasting results. Effective treatment cannot be pursued on a hit-or-miss basis; it must be directed and site specific. The common trial-and-error and shotgun therapies are destined to yield too many trials, too many errors, and very little bang for your effort.

The one thing you don't want to do with directed stretching is cause additional injury or trauma. Don't start directed stretching until you can do it without severe stabbing or shooting pain. As you will see when the specific stretches are presented in chapter 6, identifying the exact site for directed stretching is a bit more difficult than it was with targeted massage. You'll begin with some general and gentle stretching, and then you'll attempt to find the exact stretch and position that causes the greatest localized or site-specific strain. Most likely there will be one movement or stretch that actually reproduces your symptoms, and when you have found that position, you have identified the adhesion that needs to be stretched. It is vital not to cause any injury, so a gradual, slow, and steady approach is the way to begin. Fast, jerky, or bouncing motions may provide some relief, but in the long run they can do more harm than good. Just as targeted massage will get better and longer-lasting results than general massage, directed stretching will get better and longer-lasting results than general stretching. Chapter 6 will illustrate and describe various spinal stretches in detail, and you will be shown how to make each stretch specific to your needs.

Here is a simple analogy that can help you understand how targeted massage and directed stretching work best together. Imagine it's the end of summer and you've just been given a box of saltwater taffy chunks that has been sitting on the shelf since April. Chances are most of the taffy is fine, but a few chunks may be dried out and not as pliable as they were four months earlier. Their taste is just as sweet, but their consistency is a little tough. Obviously, it is unnecessary to soften (massage and stretch) the whole box when only a few chunks are rigid (in spasm). So first you need to identify the rigid (tight) taffy. Now, if you've ever had a chunk of really hard taffy, you'll know that it's almost impossible to start pulling it apart to soften it unless you've first given it a good hard smash (targeted massage). This loosens the adhesive bonds in the taffy, and now you can start to pull and stretch it to the consistency of your liking. Targeted massage will loosen the adhesive bonds in your muscles, and directed stretching will reorient the new connections into a stronger, more pliable form.

Think Back

Muscular pain is responsible for the largest percentage of neck and back pain complaints. It is primarily caused by chemical and mechanical adhesions in the muscles or connective tissue fibers. These adhesions and spasms restrict movement, irritate nerves and inhibit normal nerve impulses, reduce blood and oxygen flow, and allow the buildup of waste products, all of which causes continuous pain impulses. Targeted massage and directed stretching are the therapeutic "smart bombs" that focus directly on the specific sites of the adhesions and spasms. Targeted massage seeks to disrupt adhesions and spasms, and directed stretching seeks to restore normal movement in the site. Together they collapse the physical cycles that produce chronic muscular neck and back pain.

If all neck and back pain were caused by muscular problems, then targeted massage and directed stretching would put you well on your way to being pain free. But some neck and back pain can be caused by joint and disc problems, so you should know how to address and treat those situations too. The next chapter will discuss the causes and treatments of joint and disc pain.

CHAPTER 5

Disc and Joint Pain

If you're like most people with back pain, your greatest worry is that your condition is caused by a catastrophic joint or disc problem that will result in permanent pain or disability. The truth is that 40 percent of normal, pain-free adults have degenerative joint disease and herniated discs (Jensen et al. 1994), and only a small percentage of neck and back pain sufferers will ever have to undergo surgical corrections. And although joint and disc problems can cause significant pain, most respond very well to conservative, noninvasive treatments. After muscle strain and sprain injuries, *degenerative joint* or *disc disease* (DJD or DDD) and herniated discs (HNP, or *herniated nucleus pulposus*) are the most common diagnoses for neck and back pain. What is so interesting about these diagnoses is that while millions of people complain every day about disc degeneration and herniations, millions more have the exact same conditions with absolutely no symptoms whatsoever (Savage, Whitehouse, and Roberts 1997). Once assumed to be severe and debilitating conditions, DDD and HNP are in many cases now seen as a normal function of aging, with most patients continuing to lead active, athletic, and highly functioning lives.

PAIN PRODUCTION IN JOINTS AND DISCS

The mechanisms that produce disc and joint pain are similar to those of muscle pain. When discs and joints are functioning properly, they constantly produce a wealth of positioning and movement information and send it to the spinal cord and brain. The abundant, free flow of this information blocks pain messages in discs and joints just as it does in muscles. However, when movement becomes restricted, sensory information declines, noxious information increases, and pain occurs. Movement is the primary stimulus for blocking the production and transmission of disc and joint pain. As joint or disc movements decrease, the likelihood of pain will increase; as joint or disc movements increase, the likelihood of pain decreases.

The onset of disc or joint pain is also similar to that of muscle pain. Trauma or extended periods of limited or no movement cause disc and joint stiffness, disrupting the surrounding and supporting connective tissues. Initially, there is a period of laxity and softening of the ligaments or discs, which leads to repair by the formation of adhesive bonds and scar tissue. The elasticity that allowed for pain-free movement is replaced by rigidity and inflammation. As the process becomes more advanced, so do the destructive changes. Spinal joints are no different than other joints in your body, and when they are subjected to extraordinary forces, they can become sprained and strained, resulting in swelling, restricted movement, and pain. When the problem is not rectified early enough, joints can form bony or arthritic spurs, and discs can bulge or tear their outer rings. If the process advances too far, it will cause direct irritation of the surrounding bones, muscles, and nerves.

JOINT AND DISC PAIN PATTERNS

Unlike the localized pain that results from most muscle problems, degenerative joints and herniated discs usually have more definitive pain patterns.

Regional pain. The first pattern is a more intense form of regional pain that progresses well beyond the simple uncomfortable achiness and soreness described in chapter 4. When joint- or disc-related regional pain occurs, a severe toothlike or stabbing pain is felt almost constantly throughout the region. Then, if the combination of inflammation and restriction lasts long enough or becomes severe enough, they quickly lead to the second pattern, called referred pain.

Referred pain. This occurs when the nerves that surround your joints or discs become irritated to the point that they affect a distant area. In this situation, the pain is felt at—or *referred* to—other locations. Typically, only a small portion of a surrounding nerve is affected, so only a small portion of a distant extremity feels pain. In essence, joint or disc irritation of the surrounding nerves is stimulating or referring pain from one place to another.

Radiating pain. The last pattern of disc or joint pain is *radiating* or *radicular pain.* This

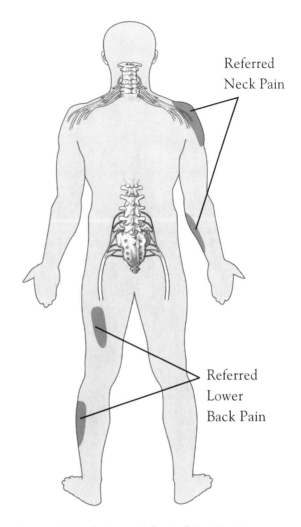

Referred Neck Pain

Referred Lower Back Pain

Figure 5.1: Referred Pain Distributions

is characterized by the same sharp, constant toothlike pain of regional joint or disc pain, but there is an additional pain that travels along the entire course of a nerve, with a constant aching, burning, numbing, and eventual weakness in the affected arm or leg. While regional pain remains in one area of the neck or back, and referred pain is felt at separate locations, radiating pain is felt throughout an entire limb. And where regional and referred pain are caused by an irritation of the smaller nerves in muscles or surrounding the spinal column, radiating or radicular pain is almost always caused by a significant inflammation or entrapment of a large spinal nerve as it exits the spinal column. The most common example of radiating pain is the unremitting leg pain

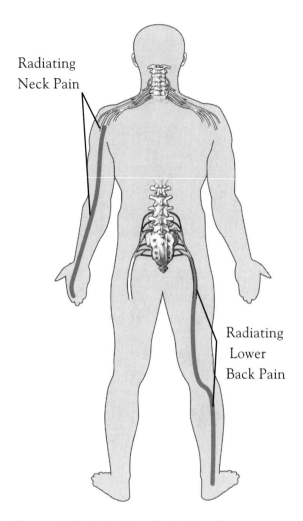

Radiating
Neck Pain

Radiating
Lower
Back Pain

Figure 5.2: Radiating Pain Distributions

called *sciatica.* One or more branches of the large sciatic nerve that run from the spinal column down into your toes is either irritated or compressed by joint inflammation, bone spurs, or a disc herniation. The nerve impingement is felt throughout the course of the nerve, all the way down to its end. The pain is generally severe and unrelenting, and if it is true sciatica pain, it can occur without any back pain at all.

Because the muscle, joint, disc, and nerve structures are so intertwined, two or more patterns can occur at one time. For example, some patients with severe regional neck or lower back pain may have a distant shoulder or calf pain too. In most of these cases, once the primary regional pain is successfully treated, the referred and radiating pain will also dissipate. Unfortunately, the reverse is not also true. When primary radiating pain is caused by direct entrapment of the spinal nerves, treating any associated regional or referred pain will have no effect on the radiating pain. The good news is that regional and referred pain are primary in most neck and back pain cases, and true spinal entrapment is a fairly rare occurrence. Consequently, if you have no obvious, severe, constant pain radiating into your arms or legs, then a conservative treatment approach directed at the simplest form of regional or referred pain is the prudent and effective place to begin.

DEGENERATIVE JOINT AND DISC DISEASE

The most common initial test used to detect degenerative disc or joint disease is a simple routine X-ray. Since 1895, X-rays have been an excellent tool for looking at bone. They are comparatively inexpensive and can usually be done right in the doctor's office. Therefore, even though X-rays are no longer considered essential unless a fracture is suspected (Agency for Health Care Policy and Research 1994; Gillan et al. 2001), many doctors still routinely X-ray patients during the first week of complaints. The result of this century-old technology and interpretation is that a large percentage show curvatures and degenerative disc or joint disease (Ehrlich 2003b), which are then offered as an explanation or diagnosis for the patient's pain. Even when treating doctors believe the joint or disc degeneration isn't significant, once patients know it exists, they are likely to believe it represents a serious neck or back problem. After

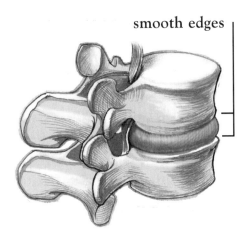

smooth edges

Figure 5.3a: Normal Disc

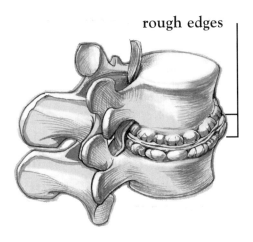

rough edges

Figure 5.3b: Degenerative Disc

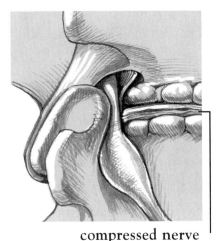

compressed nerve

Figure 5.3c: Degenerative Disc with Nerve Root Compression

all, if not put in the context of its importance, the black-and-white picture of your spine allegedly breaking down right before your eyes can be a very powerful image. And besides, if the doctor wasn't too concerned, why did she take an X-ray, and if it's not too serious, why did the X-ray show a degenerative condition?

To understand what DJD and DDD mean to you, it will be helpful to first understand what it means to the general population. It has long been established that these conditions exist in the normal, pain-free population (Kauppila et al. 1998). As a matter of fact, they appear at the same rates in the normal population as they do among people with neck and back pain. It is estimated that by age forty, 80 percent of men and 65 percent of women will show moderate degenerative changes (Miller, Schmatz, and Schultz 1988). Spinal curvatures, angulated spines, and spines with reversed curves are not seen more frequently in people with pain than they are in people without pain (Murrie et al. 2003). It is also well known that DJD and DDD take years to develop. When an X-ray reveals degeneration in a spine that has had no significant pain for years, it doesn't make sense to suddenly attribute the current pain solely to the degenerated state. The widespread attribution of DJD and DDD as causative factors is inadequate and implies that in order to treat the pain, you must treat the degenerative disease. In all but a few cases, you don't have to treat the degeneration at all.

In some instances, due to trauma, repetitive motion, or lack of movement, a degenerative joint or disc can become the major site of pain. Any of these three mechanisms can cause enough swelling and inflammation to initiate the pain cycle. But because X-rays are unable to differentiate painful from nonpainful DJD, the onset, characteristics, and location of the pain often provide the best information for making the diagnosis (Borenstein et al. 2001).

History. The primary history for the onset of degenerative joint- or disc-induced pain is usually:

- pain that begins gradually or after a prolonged period of no movement

- pain that begins after a brief period of repetitive movements

- pain that starts or gets worse after minimal work or activity

Characteristics. The primary characteristics of degenerative joint- or disc-induced pain is usually:

- pain that is fairly constant or relieved only by rest

- pain that is tolerable in the morning but gets worse as the day goes on

- pain that occasionally produces a burning or tingling in a distant part of an arm or leg

Location. Degenerative joint- or disc-induced pain is usually:

- pain that is felt directly on the spine

- pain that can cover an entire region of your neck or back and also a separate, distant part of an arm or leg

While the local and regional patterns of muscle pain tend to ease with movement and lessen as the day progresses, DJD and DDD pain is aggravated by too much movement and tends to worsen as the day goes on. The most important things to remember about degenerative joint and disc disease are that they commonly occur in pain-free people and that with a gentle and proper approach to treatment, they typically respond without prolonged pain or disability.

HERNIATED DISCS

Herniated discs conjure up a whole different set of fears and dire expectations. Discs are unjustly maligned as fragile, fickle, and ineffective structures ready to slide out of position or rupture at the drop of a hat. In fact, herniated discs actually begin slowly with tiny separations in the outer rings that eventually allow the inner nucleus to push through. This process takes time, and HNPs are now considered more a degenerative process than a traumatic one. In young, normal, and healthy discs, the amount of force required to cause a herniation is so great that it is associated with the kinds of trauma that are more likely to produce bone fractures or dislocations than to cause disc herniations (Lestini and Wiesel 1989).

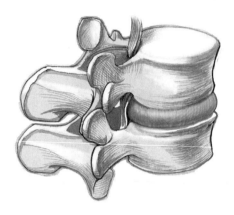

Figure 5.4a: Normal Disc

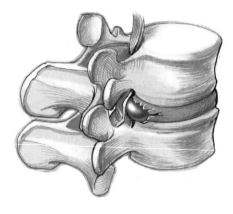

Figure 5.4b: Side View of Herniated Disc

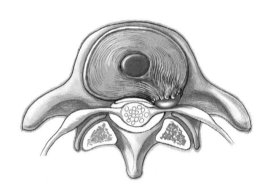

Figure 5.4c: Top View of Herniated Disc

HNPs are almost as common as degenerative joints and discs, with tens of millions of people enjoying complete, full, active, and pain-free lives never knowing they have one or more disc herniations. And just like degenerative joints and discs, HNPs are very responsive to conservative treatments, often completely or partially resolving regardless of what treatment is used (Ellenberg et al. 1983). Herniated discs are best visualized by MRI, which can provide an exquisite image of the discs and the surrounding joints, soft tissues, spinal cord, and nerves. But just as X-ray cannot show which degenerative joints are problematic, MRI cannot always show which herniations are problematic. Because MRIs reveal so many herniations in pain-free people, and HNPs respond to most conservative treatments anyway, MRI findings have little if any use in determining early therapy options (Grover and Pereira 2003). Most guidelines now call upon physicians to delay referring patients for an MRI unless there is recent, severe trauma or the patient has significant, unrelenting radiating pain for more than one month (Pettersson et al. 1997). If you are not in one of those two categories, there is a good chance your neck or back pain isn't being caused by a herniated disc.

Among adults without current or previous back pain, 33 percent have significant abnormality. Fifty-seven percent over age sixty and 20 percent under age sixty have at least one bulging disc (Boden, Davis, et al. 1990), and a major disc abnormality is seen in 14 percent of pain-free people under age forty and 28 percent of those over forty (Boden, McCowin, et al. 1990). One study showed a 35 percent abnormal rate in pain-free subjects, with patients over forty years of age having a 50 percent abnormal rate (Wiesel et al. 1984). Depending upon your age, chances are better than fifty-fifty that if you go for an MRI, some abnormality will be revealed. In a 1994 *New England Journal of Medicine* article, the author went so far as to state that "given the high prevalence of findings in [people without back pain], the discovery by MRI of bulges or protrusions in people with back pain may be coincidental" (Jensen et al. 1994, 73).

Two other well-known but rarely discussed attributes of herniated discs are their transient nature and your body's ability to remedy them. It is entirely possible that an HNP will appear one day and months later a follow-up MRI will show no evidence it ever existed. A study of forty-eight confirmed herniated discs found on follow-up that nine decreased in size by 25 percent, eight decreased in size by 50 percent, and—here is the most astounding figure— thirty-one decreased in size by 75 to 100 percent, and the largest herniations decreased the most (Maigne, Rime, and Delignet 1992). Because follow-up MRIs are seldom done in private practice, doctors usually don't get to see such dramatic results. And while it is not important to try to remember all these numbers and statistics, you should now realize that herniated discs are not the scourge they were once thought to be. Every day, your body goes about the business of healing and repairing HNPs just as it maintains every other organ, tissue, and system you have.

The first experience I had with the body's ability to heal HNPs was quite revealing. I examined a woman who had been in an automobile accident six months earlier and now had neck and back pain. She brought in MRI scans that revealed multiple disc herniations. One year later, she was in another car accident and brought in new MRIs. I was surprised to see that not only had she not sustained any new injuries, the new scans showed absolutely no evidence of the old herniations. Now don't jump to conclusions—a second car accident is no cure for the first one. But isn't it comforting to know that many herniated and bulging discs can and do resolve themselves every day?

Just like muscular pain and pain caused by degenerative joint and disc disease, herniated disc pain can often be identified by its patterns and characteristics.

History. The primary history for the onset of herniated disc–induced pain is:

- arm or leg pain that began gradually and has gotten steadily, progressively, and relentlessly worse

- arm or leg pain that began after a severe, sudden, forceful traumatic event

Characteristics. The primary characteristics of herniated disc–induced pain are:

- arm or leg pain that is constant or relieved only by rest

- arm, leg, or back pain that becomes severe as soon as you stand upright

- arm or leg pain that produces a constant burning or numbing sensation

Location. The primary location of herniated disc–induced pain is:

- from your spine through your entire arm or leg, with or without neck and back pain

If you've had an MRI and been told your problem is a herniated or bulging disc, but there hasn't been unrelenting radiating pain, numbness, or weakness, it is very possible the disc isn't the cause of your problem. And, even when a disc herniation or bulge is present, unless you have constant significant pain and weakness in your arms or legs, the prognosis for recovery with conservative treatment is excellent. In rare instances, when bone or disc degeneration becomes severe enough to dramatically narrow a spinal opening (a condition known as *spinal* or *foraminal stenosis*) or a disc herniation becomes large enough, relentless pressure can be put on the spinal cord or spinal nerve roots. This condition is characterized by almost constant pain in one or both arms or legs with numbness, tingling, and loss of strength. If you've had an MRI that confirms nerve compression at a level that corresponds to these unrelenting symptoms, and the regional neck or back pain is still present, conservatively treating the neck and back pain first may alleviate the radiating pain as well. However, if the severe arm or leg symptoms exist without any neck or back pain, then aggressive and invasive treatment may be required (Atlas and Nardin 2003). Chapter 7 will provide additional information about these treatments.

Understanding how DJD and HNPs develop, knowing their signs and symptoms, and realizing how frequently they occur in the normal, pain-free population should take much of the mystery and fear out of dealing with these problems. This information will also help you understand how and why the following treatments work and reassure you that your condition can be improved.

CONSERVATIVE TREATMENTS FOR JOINTS AND DISCS

When the hinge function of joints and the weight-distribution properties of discs come together, they form *vertebral motor units,* with each responsible for a fraction of the load and a fraction of the movement. You already know that if a joint or disc becomes injured, it will weaken, stiffen, and show degenerative changes, but interestingly enough, the reverse may also be true. Increased movement in the joints and discs works to loosen, strengthen, and slow degenerative changes. This restorative movement is best accomplished through small, incremental steps that slowly and gently rehabilitate joint and disc mechanics. Picture a rusty gate hinge. By slowly and gently working the hinge back and forth, you can gradually increase its range of opening and closing. As this happens, the corroded and rusty surfaces become smoother and more polished while regaining some of their luster. With enough time the hinge may soon function without much effort, and although it may never look perfect, with regular use and maintenance it will work just fine. The same is true for your joints and discs.

Directed Range of Motion

After years of deterioration, the once smooth and glassy surfaces of your joints and discs have become jagged, rough, dried out, and inflamed. Worst of all, they have lost the movement that is vital to their health and without which they will continue to deteriorate. By gradually, slowly, and tenderly working joints and discs back and forth through limited, comfortable ranges of motion, you can accomplish several important goals.

- The sensory nerves stimulated by movement begin to counter the pain-producing nerve messages associated with stiffness.

- Rigid, weak, and inelastic connective tissues become stronger and more flexible.

- Rough and dried-out surfaces get smoother and more lubricated, and degenerative changes will slow or in some instances even stop.

- Best of all, as function becomes increased, the swelling, inflammation, and pain are reduced.

The movements designed to gently restore joint and disc function are called *directed range of motion* exercises, and they differ from directed stretching in a fundamental way. Where directed stretching is designed for vigorous pulling of the muscle to reorient connective tissue fibers, directed range of motion is designed to slowly rehabilitate joint and disc mechanisms with gentle, tender, and comfortable movement. As with that rusty hinge, the more slow and careful movement you produce, the more range of motion you will ultimately achieve. The key to maintaining healthy joints has always been movement, and the key to restoring movement is a slow, gentle, and comfortable action between the surfaces.

The great advantage of directed range of motion exercises over other therapies is the convenience and ease with which they can be done. The mere fact that other programs require you to take a half-hour to forty-five-minute block of time out of your day restricts your ability to follow through consistently and limits their benefit. Restoring and rehabilitating joints and discs requires corrective movements done regularly throughout the day, not regularly at 7:30 each morning. In chapter 6, I'll describe and illustrate directed range of motion exercises in great detail, and you will see how you can reha-bilitate your joints and discs wherever and whenever you choose to.

Spinal Manipulative Therapy

While there are several other programs and techniques that are designed to increase joint movements, only *spinal manipulative therapy* (SMT) has gone through rigorous, controlled studies and been proven to favorably affect patient outcomes. Using carefully applied, gentle forces, spinal manipulation strives to increase motion in restricted joints that will stimulate sensory nerves and block the production of pain. SMT has also been associated with the release of the body's own natural painkillers, endorphins. Studies have shown that SMT is an appropriate, safe, and effective therapy for joint and disc pain (Agency for Health Care Policy and Research 1994). Almost all physician treatment guidelines for neck and back pain now give SMT a favor-able rating but caution that it should be performed only by a well-trained and experienced practitioner, usually a chiropractor or specialized physical thera-pist. Years ago, some doctors and patients were skeptical about the safety and effectiveness of manipulation, but it is now widely embraced. If the directed range of motion exercises in the next chapter are not sufficient in restoring pain-free movement, consider trying SMT. Chapter 7 will guide you in finding a qualified and capable practitioner of SMT and other helpful therapies.

Think Back

With more than 40 percent of normal, pain-free adults showing X-ray and MRI evidence of degenerative joint disease and herniated discs, it is now widely recognized that these findings are not necessarily synonymous with pain and debilitation. In fact, herniated and bulging discs respond very well to conservative treatments, frequently resolving without chronic or ongoing complications. Only 5 percent of pain sufferers—those who exhibit the unre-mitting radiating pain patterns of nerve entrapment—should ever have to undergo spinal surgery to correct their problem.

There is a long-standing debate among researchers as to exactly which structures are responsible for most neck and back pain. Some believe muscles are the primary source, and others favor joints and discs. The reason this debate exists is an underlying assumption that if a single cause can be identified, then a single effective treatment can be prescribed. This is a virtuous goal, but because of the complex, interconnected nature of your muscles, joints, and discs, a universally effective treatment remains impractical and elusive. For this reason, any comprehensive attempt to resolve chronic neck or back pain must include gentle and patient-specific directed range of motion exercises for joints and discs. Chapter 6 will show you exactly how to perform these exercises and how to make them specific to your condition.

Directed Range of Motion Exercises and Directed Stretching

On the most basic level, neck and lower back pain usually result from one of two things: something you've been doing to yourself or something you are not doing for yourself. In either case, your daily routine has contributed to a chronic condition desperately in need of change. Physically, your spine is composed of just flesh and bones that are constantly changing and adapting to the forces of their environment. Unfortunately, if you have neck or back pain, those adaptations have taken a restrictive and painful configuration. Tightness and adhesions have caused alterations in tissue shape and consistency, and nothing less than stopping or reversing those changes will produce lasting results. It is time to provide the proper setting for nature's adaptive process to create a looser and nonpainful spine.

In clinical practice, it is easy to distinguish patients who work at changing this process by faithfully doing their exercises from those who don't. The benefits from the work that goes into this program are so obvious that the results speak for themselves. If you had a life-threatening disease that required daily medication, you wouldn't think twice about taking your medicine. Now you have to adopt that same attitude toward your spinal exercise program. In this chapter, you will find the recommendations that are to become your daily medicine for your neck and back. And although it may sound harsh, it is fair to say that if you cannot commit to putting in the time and effort required to make long-term changes, you are probably wasting your time.

It is widely recognized that daily stretching and exercise are the best tools for stopping and reversing the detrimental changes that have already occurred. Just as bodybuilders must put in the time and effort to change the shape and consistency of their muscles, you too are going to have to spend some time and effort to change the shape and consistency of your muscles and the flexibility of your joints.

The two components of the program are directed stretching exercises and directed range of motion exercises. Directed stretching is designed to loosen and reorient muscle and connective tissues to resolve the local and regional pain discussed in chapter 4. Consequently, if your primary symptom is local or regional pain, start with and concentrate on the directed stretching exercises. The range of motion exercises are designed to slowly and progressively loosen restricted joints that cause the referred or radiating pain discussed in chapter 5. Therefore, if your primary symptoms are referred or radiating pain, start with and concentrate on the directed range of motion exercises, and postpone the stretching until your ranges of motion are increased to more comfortable levels. However, given the complex interaction of all the spinal structures, it is always a good idea to do some stretching after your range of motion exercises or some gentle range of motion exercises after your stretching. Most people with chronic neck and back pain will have a combination of tight muscles and restricted joints. And because the joints are more sensitive than the larger, broader muscles, it is a good idea to loosen the joints first.

DIRECTED RANGE OF MOTION EXERCISES

It is always prudent to begin in a slow and measured manner. Never move, stretch, or turn in a bouncing, sudden, or jerking motion, and you will likely never have a problem with any of these exercises. Try to do too much too soon, and you run the risk of causing additional injury or aggravating an existing problem. As with all treatments, the primary and overriding concern is to do no harm. Keep that in mind, and you will keep out of trouble. Directed range of motion exercises are not stretching, and if done correctly they shouldn't cause any sharp pain. If they do, or if you feel worse the following day, then they should be stopped.

It is also important not to combine bending, turning, or leaning motions into one continuous movement. For example, rolling your head around as if it were on a bobble-doll spring is unwise, may cause unnecessary strain, and is probably counterproductive. Performing any of the neck exercises in a rapid or uncontrolled manner may also make you feel light-headed or dizzy. If those symptoms persist with gentle movements, stop the exercises and consult with your physician. These procedures are designed to slowly restore movement, gently loosen adhesions, and gradually repolish surfaces. They are not aerobic activities or sporting events. Slow and steady is the key to success.

Lastly, for many patients the neck exercises will elicit a grinding, clicking, or sandpapery noise coming from your neck. Don't get upset. These noises are extremely common, and nothing is being crunched, ground, broken, or chipped away. Initially, as your range of motion increases, so may the noises. After several days of doing the exercises, and as the ranges of motion become smoother and more complete, the noises will begin to diminish and eventually may disappear altogether.

There are six basic directions or ranges of motion your neck and back can move through.

- *flexion* (downward or forward bending)

- *extension* (upward or backward bending)

- *right rotation* (turning to the right)

- *left rotation* (turning to the left)

- *right lateral flexion* (bending to the right)

- *left lateral flexion* (bending to the left)

Directed range of motion exercises begin with slow and deliberate movements in one simple direction, stopping as soon as you feel any pain, tightening, or discomfort. At that point, you will slowly return to a neutral position facing forward, and then gently repeat the movement several times in one direction, each time extending the range by just a few limited and comfortable degrees. By the third or fourth repetition, you will notice that the range increases on its own with hardly any effort on your part. After five to seven repetitions in one direction, you will repeat the procedure in the opposite direction. For example, if you have just completed five neck rotations to the right, you'll then do five gentle neck rotations to the left, again stopping at neutral after each repetition. The rotation series is then completed with five repetitions turning fully and comfortably from right to left without stopping.

Review the illustrations before starting the exercises, and keep the rusty hinge analogy in mind. Slow and gentle movements can and will restore proper joint function.

Cervical Spine (Neck) Ranges of Motion

Directed neck range of motion exercises take only five minutes and should be done at least two to three times daily or any time you are keeping your head and neck in the same position for a long time (for instance, while reading or working at the computer). Even doing a few abbreviated movements at the computer or while watching TV will help prevent stiffness from occurring or old adhesions from reforming.

FLEXION AND EXTENSION

All the neck exercises are performed sitting in an erect and upright posture looking straight ahead (neutral position). To begin the first exercise, forward flexion, let your head come slowly and gently downward with your chin tucking slightly in toward your chest. You should feel as though gravity is easing your head downward, not like you are forcing it forward. Go as far as you comfortably can, and when you feel tightness or pulling in the back of your

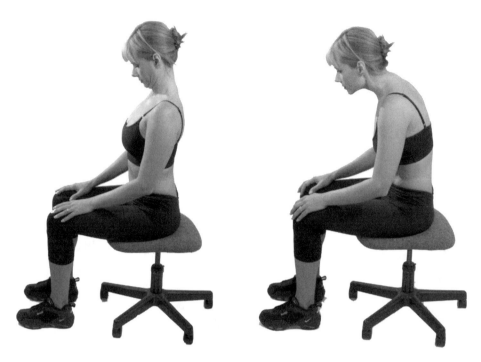

Figure 6.1a: Proper Neck Flexion   Figure 6.1b: Improper Neck Flexion

neck or upper back, stop and hold that position for three to five seconds, and then slowly come back to the neutral position. Complete five to seven of these gentle repetitions, each time trying to notice a slight increase in the overall movement. In very rare instances of severe spinal cord impingement, this exercise may cause a numbing or tingling sensation in the arms or hands. If this occurs, discontinue the exercise and consult a physician.

For cervical spine extension, sit in the same neutral position, and slowly and in a very controlled manner, allow your head to move backward. At the same time, gently elevate your chin as if you are looking up at the ceiling. Move as far as you comfortably can, and as soon as you feel any compression or pinching at the base of your head or the base of your neck, stop and slowly come back to the neutral position. Complete five to seven repetitions, each time trying to notice a slight overall increase in the ease and range of the movement. If light-headedness or dizziness occurs, you may be moving too fast, and you will have to slow the routine. If these symptoms occur with very slow and gentle movement, discontinue the exercise.

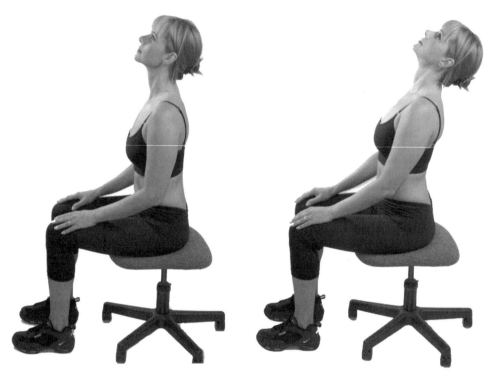

Figure 6.2a: Proper Neck
Extension

Figure 6.2b: Improper Neck
Extension

After you have finished flexion and extension, it is time to combine them into one smooth and continuous movement. Start with forward flexion, moving your head only as far forward and downward as is comfortable. From that position, carefully move your head and neck backward to a comfortable extension range, and then repeat the full cycle. This is just like gesturing yes, nodding your head fully forward and backward. This exercise opens and closes the joints in your spine like an accordion, increasing range of motion and decreasing pain. Gently complete the entire cycle five to seven times. Again, don't be concerned about any grinding or clicking noises. When the movement becomes easier, the noises will dissipate.

ROTATION

For neck rotation (side-to-side turning), start from the neutral position and slowly turn your head as if you are trying to look over your shoulder. Turn only as far as you comfortably can. When you feel tightness or pulling on the opposite side, or compression and pinching on the side you're turning toward, stop and hold that position for three to five seconds, then slowly come back to the neutral position. Repeat this five to seven times, trying to notice a slight increase in the movement with each repetition. Next, move your head in the opposite direction and gently complete another five to seven repetitions in the same manner. Once you have performed rotation to both sides, combine them into one smooth motion. This is similar to shaking your head no. Gently complete the entire cycle five to seven times.

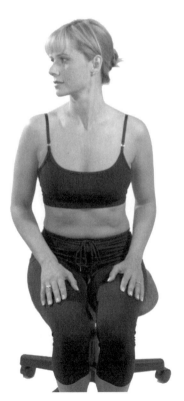

Figure 6.3a: Proper Neck Rotation

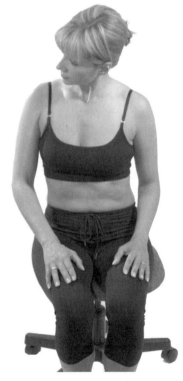

Figure 6.3b: Improper Neck Rotation

LATERAL BENDING

For side bending or lateral flexion of the neck, gently lean your head to one side as if you were trying to touch your ear to the base of your neck on the same side. Lean only as far as you comfortably can. Do not try to touch your ear as far out as your shoulder. Leaning your head too far out to one side will probably cause muscle strain on the opposite side and will not increase any joint movement. Ideally, you want to keep the center of your head over the center of your spine. When you feel any tightness or pulling on the opposite side, or compression and pinching on the same side, stop and hold the position for three seconds. Slowly return to the neutral position. Repeat five to seven times, trying to notice a slight increase in the movement with each repetition. Then carefully lean your head in the opposite direction and gently complete another five to seven repetitions in that direction. Finally, finish the side-to-side bending series by slowly combining the two movements.

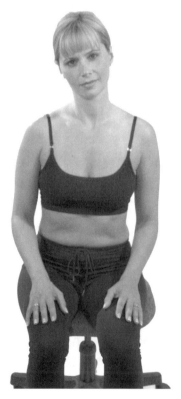 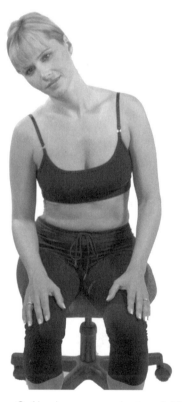

Figure 6.4a: Proper Lateral Neck Bending

Figure 6.4b: Improper Lateral Neck Bending

Lumbar Spine (Lower Back) Ranges of Motion

The lumbar ranges of motion are also designed to gently and comfortably restore lower back movement without stretching or straining the muscles. These exercises are carried out in much the same way the cervical ranges were. However, because the hips and pelvis are responsible for a significant amount of lower back bending, they must be stabilized before you can fully isolate movement to the joints of the lumbar spine. Therefore, you will also perform your lumbar ranges of motion sitting at the front edge of a firm seat.

FLEXION AND EXTENSION

Start by sitting up as straight as you can, raising your shoulders as high as possible, extending your abdomen forward, and placing a forward arch in your lower back. Keep your shoulders directly over your pelvis, and do not lean forward or backward. You should now be sitting in a military "attention" posture with a C-curve in your lower back. This is full lumbar extension (see figure 6.5a). If moving into this posture causes you to feel a compression or pinching of the spine or muscles, relax the position a little. Hold that posture for three to five seconds. When you are sitting up as straight as possible, slowly move into lumbar flexion by simply relaxing the arch in your back and allowing your chest and shoulders to gently slump downward in the direction of your lap, not outward toward your knees. Perform this downward movement while tenderly reversing the arch in your back with as little forward or backward lean as possible (see figure 6.6a). When you feel any tightness or pulling, stop and hold that position for three to five seconds, sit straight up again into lumbar extension, and then repeat the procedure five to seven times. At the end point of lumbar flexion, you should be in a hunched position and feel as though your spine is gently rounding or curving backward and downward in a reversed C posture. Complete five to seven cycles of lumbar flexion and extension, each time trying to notice a slight increase in the ease and overall range of movement. You can also do a variation of this exercise on your hands and knees by producing a lower back arch like an angry cat (flexion) and then slowly moving into a lower back dip (extension) like a swayback horse (see figures 6.7a and 6.7b).

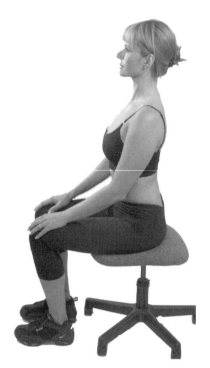
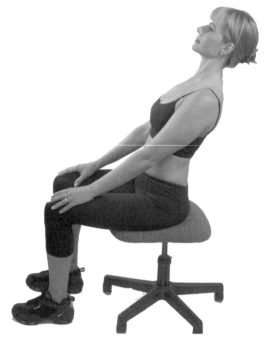

Figure 6.5a: Proper Lumbar
Extension with C-Curve

Figure 6.5b: Improper Lumbar
Extension

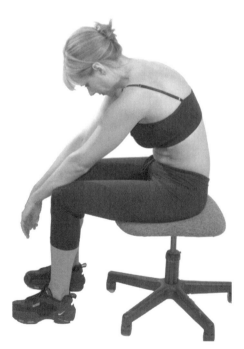
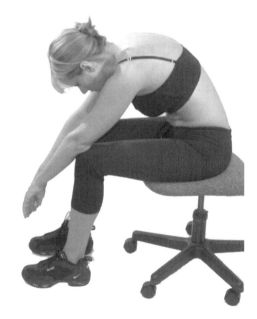

Figure 6.6a: Proper Lumbar
Flexion with Reversed C-Curve

Figure 6.6b: Improper Lumbar
Flexion

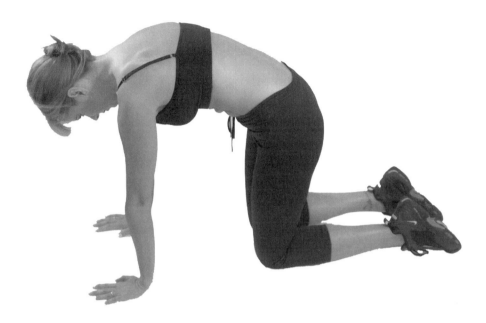

Figure 6.7a: Lumbar Flexion on Hands and Knees (Arched Back)

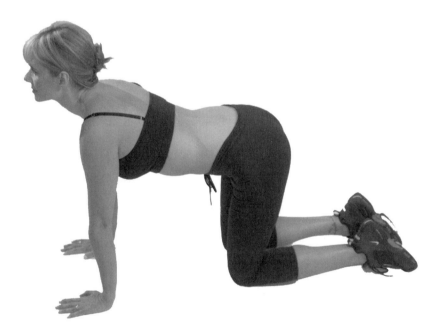

Figure 6.7b: Lumbar Extension on Hands and Knees (Swayback)

ROTATION

For lumbar rotation, start from the forward-facing seated position. Slowly turn your chest and shoulders as if you are trying to look behind you. Turn only as far as you comfortably can, and be sure not to lean to the side as you turn. When you feel tightness or pulling on the opposite side, or compression and pinching on the same side, stop and hold that position for three to five seconds before coming back to the neutral position. Repeat this five to seven times, trying to notice a slight increase in the movement with each repetition. Keep in mind that you are not trying to stretch the muscles of your lower back, you are only trying to get some gentle movement in the joints. Then turn your chest and shoulders in the opposite direction, carefully completing another five to seven repetitions. Once you have finished the rotation exercise to each side, you can combine them into one smooth motion. Gently complete the entire cycle five to seven times.

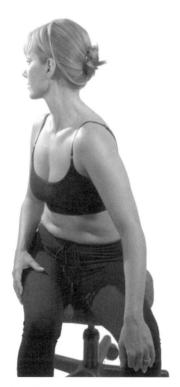 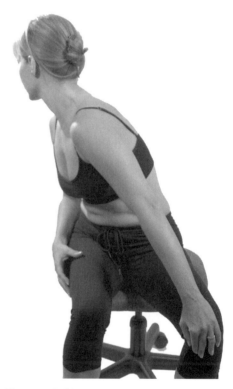

Figure 6.8a: Proper Lumbar Rotation

Figure 6.8b: Improper Lumbar Rotation

LATERAL BENDING

The joint structures of the lumbar vertebrae allow for very limited side bending, so there is no need to force this movement. Begin in the seated upright position, and gently lean your right shoulder straight down toward your right hip. Do not lean out away from your body, since this may cause muscle strain and will not increase any joint movement. Again, lean only as far as you comfortably can, and when you feel tightness or pulling on the opposite side, or compression and pinching on the same side, stop and hold that position for three seconds. Then come back to the neutral position and repeat the procedure five to seven times. Just as with the other procedures, try to notice a slight increase in the movement with each repetition. Finally, lean your left shoulder straight down toward your left hip, gently complete another five to seven repetitions to the left, and then combine the movements into a gentle and fluid side-to-side bending motion.

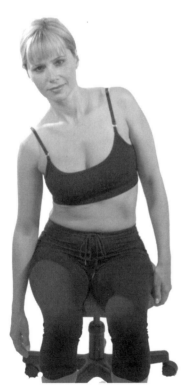
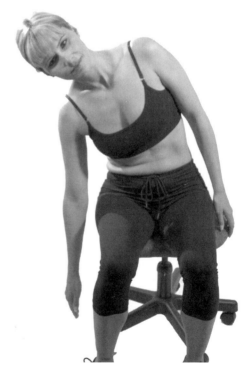

Figure 6.9a: Proper Lateral Lumbar Bending

Figure 6.9b: Improper Lateral Lumbar Bending

Although these directed range of motion exercises seem so simple, almost to the point of having hardly any therapeutic value, when you perform them conscientiously, they will become the foundation for regaining and maintaining your healthy spine.

DIRECTED STRETCHING EXERCISES

It only takes ten to fifteen minutes a day to complete a directed stretching and exercise routine, but three minutes in the morning shower will not make a dent in the process. Waking up with increased neck or back pain is a common complaint because a lack of movement at night causes stiffness in the muscles and joints. Minimal morning stretching will loosen the prior night's restrictions, but don't expect it to accomplish anything more than that. Unless you spend the necessary time to make significant and lasting changes, the cycle of chronic pain will remain unbroken.

Directed stretching can be done anywhere and any time you have fifteen minutes to yourself. Morning, afternoon, or evening, it makes no difference. If you'd like to stretch while you're watching the evening news and sipping a glass of wine, that's great. If you prefer to stretch while watching baseball and drinking beer, that's fine too. Just make sure the seventh inning stretch goes the entire inning and not just for the two-minute Budweiser commercial. The results are not dependent upon when or where you do it; the only thing that matters is how you do it. It is amazing how many millions of people freely relinquish their time, their money, and their care to modestly effective therapies that require them to travel back and forth for treatment, taking up several hours a week. By spending the same total time—or less—with a more convenient and effective home approach, you can achieve similar or better results.

Directed stretching is specifically designed to isolate and loosen the offending muscle spasms and adhesions, and to achieve the same benefits for the muscles that directed ranges of motion did for the joints. The procedures are similar in that only slow, steady, and gradual advances are recommended. However, the greater elasticity of muscles compared to joints requires increased stretching, which may be a little uncomfortable in the beginning. In fact, you'll know you've focused on the right muscle bundle when the slow and steady stretch produces a localized pain similar to the pain you felt during deep massage.

Unlike general stretching techniques that achieve only general results, directed stretching must be site specific to be effective. And, because every person is different, every person's stretching techniques will also be different. It is impossible for a broad range of general stretches to have the same beneficial effect for everyone. However, if you learn how to modify some basic stretches, they become specific to you, and your chances at a better outcome are greatly increased. The following pages illustrate how directed stretching exercises should be performed, and you will learn how to modify them for your best results.

Directed Stretching for the Neck

The aim of directed stretching for the neck is to find the position that most closely reproduces your symptoms and then target those muscles. While the joint range of motion exercises never combined flexion and extension with rotation or lateral bending, these muscle stretches will likely require a combination of movements to pinpoint the offending spasms. In order to develop the best stretch for your neck, sit upright and begin with gentle forward bending. When you feel a significant amount of pulling in the back or down the side of your neck, stop and then slowly rotate your chin from one side to the other to determine which causes more additional pulling. For example, if your neck pain is predominately on the right, slowly and gently bend your head forward until you feel a strong pulling sensation in the back or right side of your neck. Then, with your neck in the flexed position, slowly rotate your chin from left to right to see which causes more pulling, and then hold your chin in that position.

The last step in modifying this stretch is to lean your head toward the shoulder that causes the most additional pulling. Usually, if the pain is on your right side, you'll need to lean your head toward your left shoulder, and if the pain is on the left, you'll need to lean toward the right shoulder. This will produce additional pulling and stretching of the offending muscles. At this point, you should feel some very strong pulling from the side of your neck into the same side of your upper back and possibly to the shoulder blade. You have now combined flexion, rotation, and lateral bending to isolate the problematic

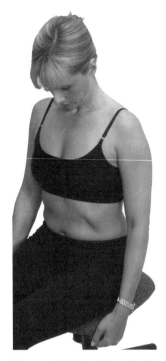

Figure 6.10a: Cervical Flexion Pulling Patterns

muscle tightness. In all likelihood, this is the exact same spot that was tender during the massage techniques.

Hold the stretch for ten to twenty seconds, and then very gently, carefully, gradually, tenderly, and cautiously move your head and neck back to the neutral position. The first time you do this, you are going to feel a significant amount of strain and pulling in the muscle, so don't force it. As you repeat this stretch seven to ten times, each repetition should bring some additional movement, relaxation, and stretching of the area. Never use your hands or any other devices to try to force or enhance the stretch. These are relatively fine muscles, and if you try to externally force the stretch, you run the risk of causing additional muscle strains and sprains.

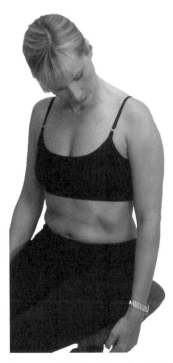

Figure 6.10b: Cervical Flexion and Rotation Pulling Patterns

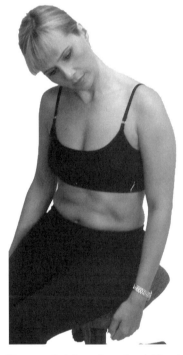

Figure 6.10c: Cervical Flexion, Rotation, and Lateral Bending Pulling Patterns

Directed Stretching for the Upper Back

As you'll recall from the targeted massage section, your neck muscles are significantly influenced by the muscles of your upper back, so it is vital to stretch these muscles too. To begin, bend your arms in at the elbows, then raise both elbows at your sides to about shoulder level. Next, slowly bring both elbows as far behind you as possible, as if you were trying to touch them together. Hold the stretch for ten to twenty seconds. This should cause a mild to moderate pain along the upper back and a feeling of squeezing or compression on the inside edges of the shoulder blades. These are large, broad muscles, so don't be afraid to give them a slow, steady, and forceful stretch. At the end of the stretch, gently bring both elbows forward and wrap your arms around your chest as if you were attempting to give someone a bear hug. Repeat the procedure seven to ten times, using a bit more force and trying to stretch a little further each time. You can make this stretch site specific by raising or lowering your elbows. If you want to feel the stretch higher on your upper back, raise your elbows. If you want to feel it further down your spine, lower your elbows.

A common variation of this stretch is to stand in a doorway, place your hands against the jambs, and then lean into the opening or push against the doorway. I do not recommend this technique. Your upper body weight is being used to force or enhance the stretch to the point where it can cause additional unintended strain.

Directed neck and upper back stretching must be done at least

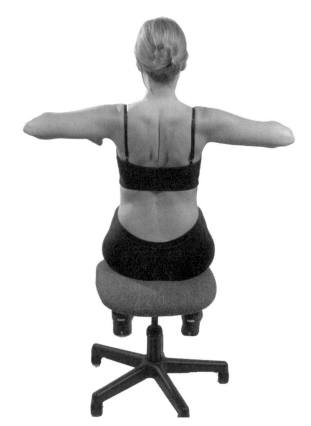

Figure 6.11: Upper Back Stretch

once a day. Take the time to make sure your efforts are targeting and stretching the precise muscle spasms and adhesions. It may take a while before you feel comfortable with these stretches. You will probably have to go back and reread this section a few times until you become proficient at them.

Directed Stretching for the Lower Back

When most people think about lower back stretching, they picture an extensive routine of bending, leaning, turning, and twisting. And although that kind of stretching will decrease symptoms, unless it is site specific, it won't make any permanent changes. It is much more desirable to perform a few directed stretches that target an offending spasm or adhesion than it is to spend extended time on less effective general stretches.

The goal of directed stretching for your lower back is the same as it was for your neck: to reveal the combination of movements that most closely reproduces your symptoms. If you are unable to stand or you are in a significant amount of pain, you can do the forward-bending exercises sitting at the front edge of a chair. Otherwise, begin standing with your feet shoulder-width apart. Initially, it is okay to bend your knees, since this may help you achieve a bit more forward bending. Until you become comfortable with the stretching, you may also want to lean on the back of a chair for additional support. The first repetition of any stretch should be always be slow and gradual, adding a bit more movement with each successive stretch. Do not overdo it by trying to accomplish too much too soon.

Start by slowly rounding your back forward from your shoulders, and then eventually from your waist. The farther down you bend, the more pain or pulling you will feel. Just as with neck flexion, instead of forcing yourself to bend forward, try to relax your back as you go and let gravity do the work. This should allow you to bend a little easier and stretch a bit farther. If you reach a point where you can't possibly go any lower, or the pain is about to take your breath away, stop and hold the position for ten to twenty seconds. You may notice a strong pull in the muscles parallel to your spine and in your upper buttock. In the next two exercises, as you modify the stretch, that pull will become more directed at the offending tightness or adhesion. Now, slowly ease your way to an upright position again, leaning on a chair or bending your knees if you need to. Take a few steps around the room, and then repeat this procedure seven to ten times.

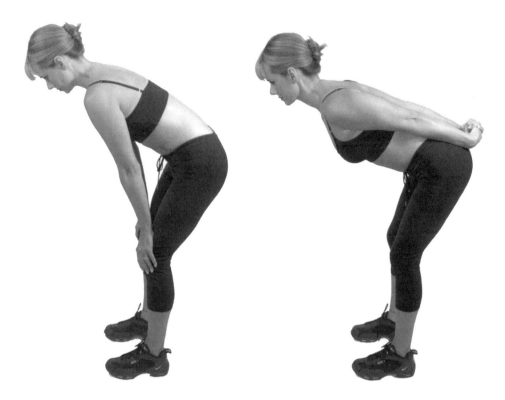

Figure 6.12: Lumbar Flexion
Pulling Pattern

Figure 6.13: Lumbar Flexion with
Hands Behind Back

You may be able to enhance stretching of the lumbar muscles by keeping your arms behind your back when you bend forward. This helps pull your shoulders back and should isolate the upper lumbar muscles.

Step two is to add some extension, or backward bending. Begin by clasping your hands in front or placing them on your hips, and take a large step forward with one leg. Keep the rear leg straight, and slowly bend your front knee so your hips begin to move forward into a gentle lunge. As the hips move forward, try to keep your shoulders directly over your hips without leaning forward or backward. This position will put a gentle C-curve into your lumbar spine, and you should feel some mild compressive pain or pressure in your lower back, along the crest of your hip. This is likely the same spot you isolated during targeted deep massage. Hold this position for ten to twenty seconds, then slowly return to a normal posture and take a few steps around the room. After seven to ten repetitions, repeat the same procedure with the other leg forward. The stretches should be slow and deliberate, gently increasing the ranges with each repetition.

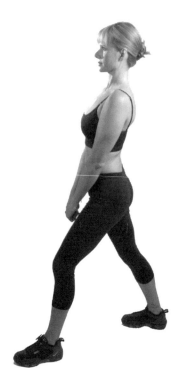

Figure 6.14a: Proper Lumbar
Extension

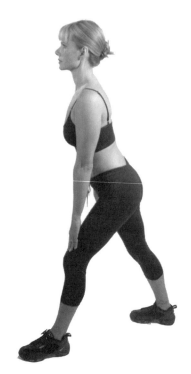

Figure 6.14b: Improper Lumbar
Extension (Shoulders Too Far
Forward)

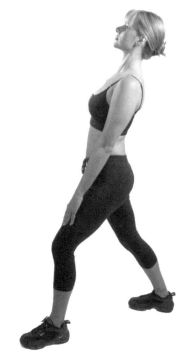

Figure 6.14c: Improper Lumbar
Extension (Shoulders Too Far Back)

After you have completed seven to ten repetitions each of forward and backward bending, it is time to move on to the next step, the addition of rotation and lateral bending. A strong word of caution is necessary here. These are compound movements that should always be done with great care. The maximum stretch is achieved with deliberate patience and good technique. Rushed or sloppy stretching will be ineffective and may be counterproductive.

To fully target your lumbar stretch, bend as far forward as possible using the same technique described for lumbar flexion. Once you have reached the maximum stretch, slowly and gently reach one of your hands to the opposite ankle: left hand to right ankle or right hand to left ankle, whichever more closely reproduces your symptoms. It is okay to bend at the knees a bit, and doing so may increase your stretch. These movements are a combination of lumbar rotation and lateral bending, and the key to making this specific to your condition is in finding the amount of flexion, rotation, and lateral bending that produces the greatest amount of stretching and discomfort. When you have found that position, you have isolated the site of your problem and identified the area in

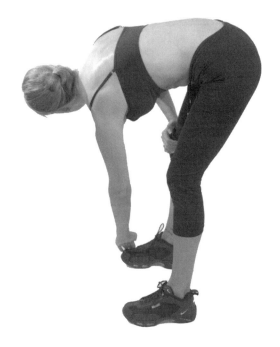

Figure 6.15: Lumbar Flexion, Rotation, and Lateral Bending

need of the most attention. As with the other stretches, slowly and gradually increase the movement with each successive repetition.

Remember that sudden, jerky, or bouncing movements are potentially harmful. From a mechanical standpoint, combined motions like these place significant stress on the spine and discs, and some critics caution against their use. But your spine, discs, and muscles are very dynamic structures with a tremendous ability to respond to these movements and forces in a positive and adaptive manner. Movement is required to disrupt old adhesions and organize the deposition of new tissue patterns. However, lifting, working, or staying in these positions for extended periods can cause excessive strain, so thirty seconds is the maximum time you want to spend in these stretches.

While doing any directed stretching, you always want to focus on increasing your movement. The gradually increasing movements will give you the positive feedback and motivation to continue. If you are focused on the pain you may be feeling, you will likely limit your stretching—and your results. Remember, these exercises are designed to identify the offending muscle, target the site for stretching, and produce changes in the shape and consistency of chronic muscle spasms. Rushing through a few stretches will never accomplish that goal. You must take your time and measure your progress not only from day to day but also from stretch to stretch.

Mirror Image Stretching

After you complete each full repetition of directed neck or lower back stretching, you are going to mildly stretch in the direct opposite or mirror image direction. For example, if you have just bent forward, turned to the right, and leaned right, you are now going to bend gently backward, turn to the left, and lean left. The initial directed stretch will loosen spasm and adhesions, and the reverse mirror image stretch will restore the gliding action between the adjoining muscle fibers. Both movements will stimulate the motor and sensory nerves that help block the production of pain.

TWO ADDITIONAL LOWER BACK STRETCHES

Here are two general stretches that are worth doing.

Knee-to-Chest Stretch

Because lower back pain is usually worse in the morning, doing a simple stretch before you get out of bed will be beneficial in reducing morning tightness. Lying flat on your back with your head on a pillow, or on one side with the lower leg slightly bent, bend your upper leg so you can grab the front of your knee with both hands. Then slowly pull your knee toward your chest. When you get to the point where you feel some moderate pulling in your lower back and upper buttock, hold that position for ten to fifteen seconds and then let go and slowly straighten your leg. Repeat this procedure seven to ten times, each time trying to bring your knee a little closer to your chest. Then repeat the entire procedure on the opposite side, pulling the other leg toward your chest. Never bring both knees toward your chest at the same time.

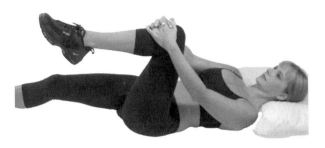

Figure 6.16a: Knee-to-Chest Stretch Lying Flat

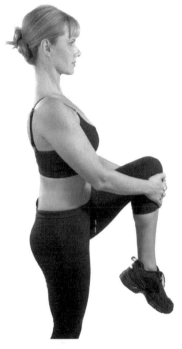

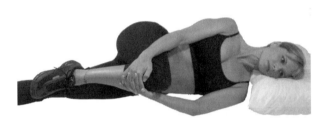

Figure 6.16b: Knee-to-Chest Stretch Lying on One Side

Figure 6.16c: Knee-to-Chest Stretch Standing

Although this simple exercise will not bring about lasting change, it is effective in temporarily relieving lower back tightness during the day or when there is no time for directed stretching. If there is no place to lie down, you can also do this exercise standing with your back against a wall.

Straight Leg Raising

The last lower back stretch, straight leg raising, is particularly effective for lower back pain accompanied by referred or radiating pain in the buttock and down your leg. This is a difficult stretch to do by yourself, and it is best if someone is there to assist. Getting help with this stretch allows you to relax the surrounding muscles and let your assistant do the work. This stretch is designed to loosen muscles in the lower back, buttock, and hamstring (back of your thigh). It can have the added benefit of decompressing the large sciatic nerve that may be entrapped or irritated by surrounding tissues and is often associated with referred or radiating leg pain.

Start by lying flat on your back on the floor, couch, or bed. Use a thin pillow to support your neck. Have your assistant reach down and grab underneath the ankle of the affected leg. Keeping your unaffected leg straight or slightly bent at the knee, have your assistant slowly start to raise the affected leg a few inches off the floor. Try to stay as relaxed as possible and let your helper do the work. This is usually a painful and difficult stretch that requires great patience and a little courage. Initially, your assistant should only raise the leg four to five

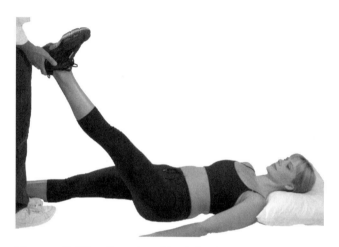

Figure 6.17a: Passive Straight Leg Raising

inches, or to a point where you feel significant pulling and stretching in your back and hamstring muscles. Have your helper hold your leg in that position for ten seconds and then gently lower it again. If necessary, take a few deep breaths, and then keep repeating this procedure, each time trying to get your straight leg raised a few inches higher. For the first two or three days, you may only get your leg to a 30- or 45-degree elevation. Within a week to ten days, you may be able to get to a 60- to 75-degree elevation without much pain.

Although straight leg raising is most effective when you can stretch passively with a helper, there are two

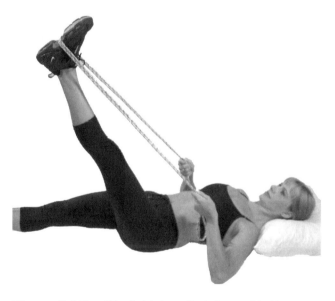

Figure 6.17b: Straight Leg Raising with Rope

variations you can try if you are by yourself. First, sitting up and holding one end of a long belt, rope, or stretch band in each hand, lean forward and place the middle of the rope on the bottom of your foot. Now lie back, and keeping your leg straight, pull on the rope to slowly elevate your straight leg off the floor. When you feel moderate pulling and stretching in your back and hamstring muscles, hold your leg in that position for ten seconds and then gently place it back on the floor. Repeat the procedure, each time trying to raise your leg a few inches farther off the

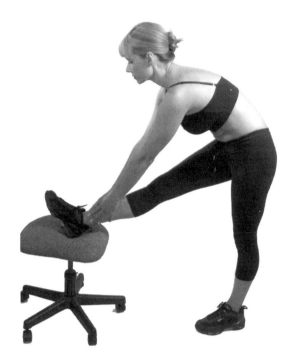

Figure 6.17c: Standing Straight Leg Raising

floor. Eventually, you should be able to raise the straight leg to a 60- to 75-degree elevation without much pain.

You can also do a straight leg stretch from a standing position by placing the heel of your foot on a stair step or a chair. Obviously, the higher you raise your leg, the more difficult the stretch will be, so you want to start out at a relatively low elevation. With the leg extended straight out, slowly and gently lean forward toward your foot. Instead of raising your leg, you are lowering your upper body. This stretches the lower back and hamstring muscles and accomplishes exactly the same goal of decompressing or freeing the entrapped sciatic nerve.

Think Back

Directed range of motion exercises and directed stretching are essential components of a home treatment program. Directed range of motion exercises are comfortable movements designed to gently restore joint motion and increase joint sensory input. They are effective for referred or radiating pain. Directed stretching helps alleviate the chronic pain cycle by providing increased movement and increased sensory information that quiets and blocks the production of pain impulses. It also helps change the shape and consistency of chronically tight tissues. Relieving your chronic neck or back pain may be a long and difficult task, but with hard work and dedicated effort, you can do it.

CHAPTER 7

Assessing Other Therapies

When targeted massage, directed range of motion, and directed stretching aren't enough to stop or reverse chronic neck or back pain, additional therapies may be necessary. Therefore, you should be aware of the range of conservative, noninvasive therapies and the more aggressive, invasive therapies that are available to you. You should also know how to evaluate the effectiveness of each therapy and how to choose the right practitioner for you.

CONSERVATIVE, NONINVASIVE THERAPIES

Conservative, noninvasive therapies—those that don't require surgeries or injections—are appropriate for 95 percent of all people with neck and back pain. Therefore, these treatments are the wise and prudent place to begin any therapy program. There is a wide selection of conservative options for neck or lower back pain, with the best known being medication, physical therapy, chiropractic, physiatry, massage therapy, acupuncture, back schools, sports medicine, and yoga. They employ tools such as diathermy, ultrasound, electrical muscle stimulation, exercise machines, manipulation, needles, general exercise, stretching, ice, and heat. From there the list goes on to unconventional treatments, including tai chi, Pilates, reflexology, Rolfing, herbal medicine, aromatherapy, and prayer. What makes these choices so interesting is that there is one for every lifestyle, and yet they all achieve about the same results. Until now, there has been no clear-cut or definitive guidance as to what constitutes effective treatment and what you should expect from the people who are treating you. This chapter will provide that guidance.

Therapy and Research Are Industries

If you want to find out what really works and what doesn't, ask other patients, not the therapists or researchers. Therapists get paid for delivering therapy, and researchers get grants and salaries to do research. Unless they come up with a therapy recommendation that promotes more therapy or a research recommendation that promotes more research, they are out of business. It's no wonder the most common therapy recommendation is more therapy and the most reported neck and back pain research finding is the need for more research. How else can you explain the fact that after all the years of increasing pain and suffering, researchers and therapists haven't been able to definitively say what works and what doesn't? All they've produced are definite maybes.

Physical therapists and sports medicine doctors would like nothing more than to be able to say that chiropractic is a sham, it doesn't work, come see us. And of course, chiropractors would equally enjoy making similar statements about physical therapists. The reason neither profession makes such remarks is not an unwritten code of mutual respect but the simple fact that neither profession can back up their position. They both get the same results, and according to several studies, neither is that much better than an educational handbook that includes general exercises (Cherkin et al. 1998; Hurwitz et al. 2002). That being said, in many cases professional help will be of great benefit in controlling symptoms, so here's what to look for and what to look out for.

Finding a Reputable Practitioner

Before choosing a treatment approach or consulting a doctor or therapist, the best recommendation you can have is a direct referral from a friend, coworker, or medical professional. This referral should come from someone who has had firsthand experience with the person they are referring you to. Because no standard treatment protocol will fit every patient, it is essential that you find a professional who will listen to you, someone you can talk to and work closely with. An open dialogue with your specialist is the only way to ensure that you'll get the right combination of procedures to maximize your results and minimize complications. You want to find someone who is realistic about what can and cannot be accomplished, someone with experience in treating symptoms like yours, and someone who will give you specific and honest answers to your questions.

The two important questions you must ask are:

What is the diagnosis? Based on what you learned in chapters 3, 4, and 5, the practitioner's response to this question should make sense to you. Your diagnosis should result from a combination of your symptoms, clinical findings, and any X-ray or MRI tests you may have had. If the doctor's diagnosis is primarily based on an X-ray or MRI, it may not accurately represent your true situation. Don't be intimidated or shy about asking follow-up questions or requesting additional explanations. The consultation time is not only for the doctor to get a sense of what your problem is, it is also a time for you to get a sense of what kind of practitioner the doctor or therapist is.

How long will it take? While no one has a crystal ball, and doctors and therapists should never guarantee results, they also should never give evasive or noncommittal responses such as "Every case is different" or "These things take time." You are not asking about most cases, you are asking about your case, and you already know that everything takes time. A knowledgeable and experienced practitioner will have specific answers. Vague and noncommittal responses show a lack of motivation and a less-than-dedicated desire to expedite your results. There may be times in your treatment when you hit roadblocks or plateaus, and if you aren't getting basic questions answered in a clear and definitive manner, chances are that professional won't be much help in uncovering or removing hidden obstacles if they arise.

ONE-ON-ONE ATTENTION

The improper use of equipment or stretching can do more harm than good, so regardless of the therapy you choose, you must make sure you get personalized attention. Someone should always be available to monitor and modify your technique. Oftentimes the largest and apparently most sophisticated settings are nothing more than high-end therapy mills, running patients through standard protocols with little regard for individual needs. And even though a large percentage of patients get results in spite of such detached care, you deserve personal attention during all procedures.

This is true even in group classes and instruction. There will be stretches, movements, or positions you won't be able to do or for that matter shouldn't do. It's essential that you consult with the instructor prior to taking classes, and class sizes should be small enough that the instructor can monitor your technique and progress. Allowing yourself to get lost in the shuffle is the quickest way to lose motivation and ultimately drop a class.

WARNING SIGNS

One sure sign you are in the wrong place is if the doctor or instructor is more concerned with their approach than they are with your results. The best example of this kind of detached treatment is if you are not making reasonable progress and are being told not to worry, just keep coming three times a week for another four weeks. Or you may be told that you need to come for treatment to prevent additional degenerative problems in the future. These statements are nothing more than self-serving sales pitches based on fear and scare tactics. Though it may be true that without regular movement, degenerative changes can occur, there has never been any proof that going for regular treatments slows or prevents that process.

Reasonable treatment recommendations begin with an initial trial course of therapy for one to two weeks. At that time your response should be assessed, and if necessary, appropriate modifications can be made. Patients aren't all the same, and they all don't need treatment three times weekly for six to eight weeks. It is important to choose someone who will not only provide quality treatment but also take on the role of educator, coach, and provider of reassurance. If you are being advised that more and more treatment is the only way out of your situation, head straight for the door and don't look back. True professionals should be looking out for your best interest before their own. A connected and concerned attitude of commitment should come across loud and clear in everything they say or do.

MEASURING PROGRESS

A good way to evaluate the effectiveness of whichever therapy you choose is by my 15-50 rule of response. If the therapy you are engaged in is appropriate and helpful, then every fifteen days you should be able to appreciate a 50 percent improvement of your condition. For example, after the first fifteen days, you should feel 50 percent better; fifteen days later, you should feel another 50 percent better (a 75 percent overall improvement after thirty days); and you should feel an 87 percent improvement after forty-five days. This is a generous yardstick, and if your therapy is not meeting these minimum levels of improvement, it is probably ineffective. Although "Do no harm" is always the first principle in any treatment regimen, "Do some measurable good" must also apply. A proficient doctor or therapist will always find the exact spots to target. And although it may take a few visits to open up communication and zero in, your results should reflect that level of dedication. Never, ever settle for general procedures or marginal results.

Home Care

Every effective therapy will provide a regimen of appropriate home care. No matter which therapy you choose, doing nothing on days you don't get treatment will prolong your symptoms and delay your recovery. A classic example is the patient who goes in for treatment three times weekly, feels modestly better after therapy, does nothing in between treatments, and shows minimal overall improvement. In this scenario, the patient will say something like "I feel better after treatment, but by the next day or two, I'm right back where I was." What's worse is the therapist who responds, "Don't worry, these things take time. Just keep coming for more treatment." If you rely on marginally effective treatments to chip away at your problem and you don't do any self-treatment at home, you will eventually become dissatisfied. You may jump from one therapy to the next, ultimately remaining disillusioned and in pain. To maximize your results, you must be doing some kind of prescribed home care.

Basic Therapy Options

Ice, heat, and medication are the simplest treatment options. You can use them alone or in conjunction with other therapies.

ICE AND HEAT

For mild to moderate neck and back pain, ice and heat both provide temporary relief of symptoms. They act as counterirritants that block the transmission of pain impulses by overloading the sensory nerves with either cold or hot sensations. In the first twenty-four hours of an acute injury, sprain, or strain, ice is preferred because it also has anti-inflammatory properties. The cold actually causes small blood vessels to narrow, and that limits the amount of swelling and irritation. In the absence of acute swelling or recent trauma, heat is preferred; it causes small blood vessels to increase in size and tight muscles to relax. This helps remove waste products from the muscle and increases the supply of oxygen and nutrients in healing tissues. See chapter 4 for instruction on the application of ice and heat.

MEDICATION

Medication is usually the first treatment people seek, and in many cases, it can be effective in relieving symptoms until healing occurs. The three basic types of medication are *analgesics,* or pain medications; nonsteroidal anti-inflammatory drugs (NSAIDs); and muscle relaxers. Analgesic and anti-inflammatory medicines are readily available in nonprescription, over-the-counter strengths. Acetaminophen, the active ingredient in Tylenol, is the most common analgesic, but it has no anti-inflammatory properties. The reasoning behind the use of acetaminophen is simple: it helps relieve pain. NSAIDs such as aspirin and ibuprofen have both analgesic and anti-inflammatory properties and are therefore usually preferred over analgesics alone. The theory behind the use of NSAIDs is to decrease any swelling or inflammation that may be contributing to the pain. Both types of medication have their side effects and disadvantages. Though it's rare, high doses of acetaminophen can cause liver damage, extensive ibuprofen use is associated with kidney damage, and NSAIDs in general are a common cause of stomach upset.

Conservative Therapies for Regional and Referred Pain

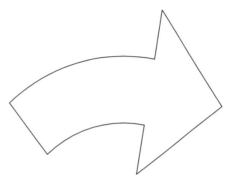

Muscle Tightness

Ice and Heat
Medication
Physical Therapy
Back Schools
Chiropractic
Acupuncture
Massage
Exercise
Yoga
Tai Chi
Pilates

Joint Stiffness

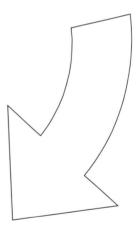

Nerve Irritation

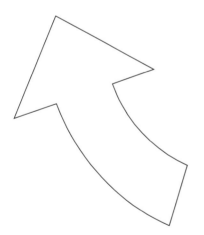

Figure 7.1: Conservative Therapies

In cases of extreme muscle tightness, muscle relaxants can be prescribed to reduce the most severe spasms. For mild to moderate spasms, muscle relaxers have not been shown to be any more effective than NSAIDs. Because muscle relaxers have a higher rate of unwanted side effects—including sleepiness, dizziness, and lethargy—their use is usually reserved for the most severe cases of spasm, and they are available by prescription only.

When you are taking any medications, it is important to read the label and heed the recommended doses. Also, you should consult with your doctor if you are taking any other medications, if you have any unwanted side effects, or if the condition is not improving within two days.

Professional Therapy Options

Let's take a closer look at some of the most common noninvasive therapies for neck and back pain.

PHYSICAL THERAPY, PHYSIATRY, REHABILITATION, AND SPORTS MEDICINE

Physical therapy, physiatry, rehabilitation, and sports medicine are probably the most conventional and widely used approaches of all neck and back pain therapies. Initially, they rely heavily on the use of pain control methods such as transcutaneous electrical stimulation, ultrasound, diathermy, electrical muscle stimulation, and heat or ice applications. *Transcutaneous electrical stimulation* (TENS) is a nerve stimulator that produces signals which block the transmission of pain impulses. In cases of severe and intractable pain, TENS may be prescribed for home use. *Ultrasound* and *diathermy* are forms of deep tissue heating that are meant to increase blood flow and stimulate tissue repair. *Electrical muscle stimulation* (EMS) is designed to help in tissue repair by stimulating low-level movement in the muscles. While these tools are widely used and often help to temporarily relieve pain, none of them are proven to speed your recovery or alter the ultimate outcome.

Physical therapy, rehabilitation, and sports medicine place a strong emphasis on a presumption that the core (internal supportive) muscles of the back and abdomen are responsible for most lower back conditions. One of their main protocols is to use machines and equipment to strengthen these muscles. This increased strength is short-lived, however, and quickly reverts back to your natural levels once the exercises are stopped. Any small increases in core muscle strength are not responsible for the reductions in pain beyond what would be achieved by a general exercise program. A typical physical therapy treatment consists of one or two of the treatments mentioned above (TENS, ultrasound, diathermy, or EMS), a few minutes of general stretching and massage, and then a thirty- to forty-five-minute strengthening routine on the various machines and equipment.

The benefits of physical therapy, rehabilitation, and sports medicine include pain control, low risk of additional injury, and short-term increases in muscle strength. The disadvantages are that these approaches have never been shown to affect the outcome, multiple weekly appointments must be kept, the treatment sessions are long, the cost of treatment is high, and patients can develop an unintended reliance on treatment. When treatment guidelines are being assessed, these therapies often receive high appropriateness ratings, but one study did find that receiving physical therapy was associated with longer periods of pain (van den Hoogen et al. 1997).

BACK SCHOOLS

Back schools are classes or meetings offered at a local gym or "Y" that provide general back pain informational booklets, group stretching programs, and home exercise pamphlets. Because they must appeal to a wide audience, their information and techniques are usually too general to significantly influence individual cases beyond what would be expected from any other general program. If the school is oriented toward educating you on the natural wonders of your spine and your body's ability to heal itself, then it may be an excellent starting point to obtain some back pain information. But overall, in controlled studies, the ability of back schools to change the outcome of your condition has not been substantiated.

CHIROPRACTIC

Chiropractic is similar to physical therapy in its application of ultrasound, diathermy, EMS, and soft tissue techniques, but it relies less heavily on strengthening equipment. Instead, chiropractic emphasizes joint movement, and treatments usually include spinal manipulation therapy or adjustments to mobilize or loosen spinal joints. (See chapter 5 for additional information on spinal manipulation therapy.) Chiropractic care is possibly the most popular and widely used nonmedical treatment. More than 10 percent of the population have used chiropractic treatment for their current neck and back pain (Eisenberg et al. 1998). Despite years of being medically ostracized, chiropractic continues to gain in popularity, satisfaction measures, and scientific credibility. The profession now enjoys a level of acceptance that makes it a mainstream primary treatment option.

The benefits of chiropractic are similar to those of physical therapy, rehabilitation, and sports medicine. They include pain control, low risk of additional injury, and short-term increases in joint movement. The disadvantages to chiropractic are multiple weekly appointments, long treatment sessions, a high cost of treatment, and the possibility of an unintended reliance that may lead to more recurrences of pain (Carey et al. 1999).

ACUPUNCTURE

Originally an ancient Chinese healing art, acupuncture has gained popularity in the United States in the last twenty years. The primary therapeutic approach involves the insertion of extremely thin needles just below the skin's surface. One theory behind the effectiveness of acupuncture is that the insertions stimulate the body to produce naturally occurring pain-relieving chemicals. Another theory sees the needles as a counterirritant that blocks the production of pain impulses. The process of needling is not painful, and most patients describe the insertion as a very light pinching sensation. Needles may be placed in and around the painful sites as well as at other points on the body that the practitioner feels will help relieve the condition. The needles usually remain in place from ten to fifteen minutes and are then removed and discarded. Some practitioners try to further stimulate the area by adding small electrical currents to the needles, or by using a cupping or suction technique to bring additional blood to the region.

A typical course of acupuncture consists of approximately ten thirty-minute treatments. Though some patients may experience slight discomfort, the treatments are considered very safe with few potential side effects. As with physical therapy and chiropractic, if the treatments are going to be successful, you should notice some significant improvement within the first few sessions, and the same 15-50 rule of response applies.

MASSAGE

The effectiveness and techniques of targeted tissue massage were extensively covered in chapters 4 and 6. Its ability to disrupt adhesions, relax muscle spasm, increase blood flow, and release natural pain blockers is well documented. General massage usually feels good, and although that is a worthwhile benefit in itself, most "relaxing" massage techniques have no proven therapeutic value. The significant advantages of massage are that it can be done at home and on your schedule, it is not time consuming, there are few side effects, and the cost is low. The disadvantages to massage include ineffective application or possible soreness of the region the following day.

Exercise-Based Therapy Options

General exercises, yoga, tai chi, and Pilates are essentially different forms of exercise that create movement for the spine and surrounding muscles. No single approach enjoys any specific advantages or benefits over the others, and because they all get the same results, choosing your method of exercise is more a matter of lifestyle preferences than anything else. The important thing is that you choose a discipline you'll feel comfortable with and one you are likely to continue with.

GENERAL EXERCISE

General exercises that improve conditioning and aerobic activity are helpful in relieving neck and back pain (Lively 2002; Moffett et al. 1999). Whether it is weight training, walking, or bicycling, exercise is an essential ingredient in every recovery program, and it may be the single best preventer of reoccurrences (Linton and van Tulder 2001). Choose the activities you like best, alternate them to prevent boredom, and then start exercising. If you have a medical condition that prohibits vigorous exercise or activity, be sure to consult a physician before beginning any program. Always start slowly and gently, building up to a routine of thirty minutes per day. Most of all, remember why you are doing this. You are not entering a beauty pageant or an endurance or strength competition. Your goal is to slowly and comfortably heal your body.

YOGA

Yoga is another ancient Eastern practice that has become very popular in the United States. Practitioners stretch into various poses and hold the positions while incorporating breathing and relaxation techniques into the stretch. Yoga does not require any special equipment, it is low cost, and it can be done at home or in group classes. While most movements can produce the beneficial effects of general stretching, you must remember not to overstretch or strain already weakened areas. The drawbacks to yoga are that it lacks specificity in targeting precise spasms and that the poses don't produce the dynamic motion that helps lay down organized tissue patterns. Nonetheless, yoga is an excellent means of regaining and maintaining good spinal movement.

TAI CHI

Tai chi is a noncombative martial art that trains its practitioners in slow, gentle, and continuous movements. Unlike the static stretching poses of yoga, the emphasis of tai chi is on fluid, dynamic joint motion. Where yoga may be more appropriate for people with muscular neck and back pain, tai chi is best suited for people with degenerative disc- or joint-induced pain. If vigorous exercise is inappropriate, or you don't enjoy taking classes at a gym, then individual or home yoga and tai chi instruction are excellent alternatives.

PILATES

Pilates is an exercise program first developed in the 1920s that is gaining newfound popularity. This approach is now being hailed as everything from a natural body sculpting miracle to the newest back pain treatment craze. The main procedure is one of rapid arm and leg movements through limited ranges of motion. The ultimate goal is increased muscle tone with a minimum of joint stress. Pilates also improves posture and balance, which may contribute to its overall benefit. Pilates holds no special benefit over other exercise programs; they are all relatively successful in producing nonspecific results through the broad effect of general exercise.

AGGRESSIVE, INVASIVE THERAPIES

In severe cases, where at least four weeks of conservative, noninvasive treatments have failed to relieve constant referred or radiating patterns of neck and back pain, more aggressive treatments may be necessary. These procedures carry the higher risks that are associated with anesthesia and infections. Generally speaking, you should not consider invasive therapies unless you have significant pain or weakness in one or both arms or legs. Additional symptoms that warrant the investigation of aggressive therapies include stabbing or shooting pain, tingling, a sensation that the extremity is falling asleep, loss of function, or an inability to easily move your limbs. Progressive weakness, numbness, decreased reflexes, or increased pain with movement are all signs of direct nerve involvement that is not being relieved by the conservative therapies. Conversely, if you don't have these signs and symptoms, it usually indicates that aggressive or invasive treatments are not warranted.

Because severe neck or back pain can have multiple causes, you want to make sure you have explored every possible conservative approach before starting aggressive treatments. If the cause of pain in an arm or leg is severe regional or referred neck or back pain, then treating the source of the pain conservatively should relieve the extremity pain as well. However, when you have arm or leg pain that continues even though your neck or back is no longer painful, then in all likelihood the pain is caused by direct spinal cord or nerve root compression that will have to be treated invasively.

The two conditions most appropriate for the use of invasive treatments are:

- disc herniations where a confirmed spinal cord or nerve root entrapment is causing neurological symptoms that correlate to the site of the herniation

- spinal stenosis, a condition in which the spinal canal or nerve root exit is narrowed by degenerative or arthritic irritation that produces symptoms that correlate to the site of the stenosis

If you have unremitting neurological symptoms that do not respond to conservative care, the following invasive treatments may be recommended.

Aggressive Therapies for Unrelenting Radiating Pain

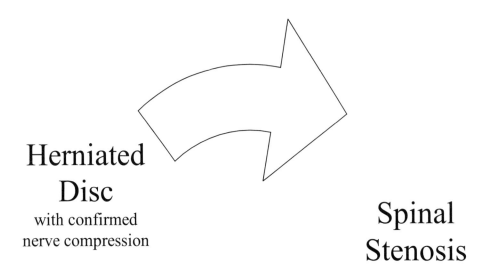

Herniated Disc
with confirmed
nerve compression

Spinal Stenosis

Epidural Steriod Injection (ESI)
Spinal Surgery
Intradiscal Electrothermal Therapy (IDET)
Radio Lesioning
Trigger Point Injections

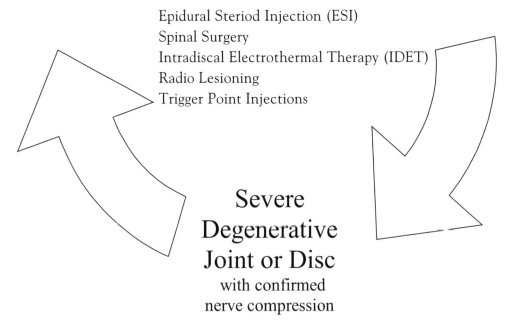

Severe Degenerative Joint or Disc
with confirmed
nerve compression

Figure 7.2: Aggressive Therapies

Epidural Steroid Injections

Epidural steroid injections (ESI) are injections into the spinal canal that are intended to reduce the swelling or inflammation of the surrounding tissues that cause nerve pain. The research reviews for this procedure offer mixed opinions. The treatment is not recommended for herniated discs, but in some cases of spinal stenosis and joint irritation, ESI is helpful in reducing inflammation and relieving symptoms for extended periods. Because canal narrowing is permanent, irritation can return, and the procedure may need to be repeated (Delport et al. 2004). ESI is usually administered as a series of three injections over a six-week period. If the first injection does not provide a modest reduction in symptoms, the treatments will probably be unsuccessful, and there is no need to undergo any additional injections.

Spinal Surgery

The most important factor in predicating a favorable surgical outcome is making sure you are the right patient for the procedure. Spinal surgery is most effective for people who have no neck or back pain but have constant radiating pain into an extremity. Surgery is never a reasonable treatment option for neck or back pain if you do not have radiating symptoms. You should wait to consider surgery until the extremity pain becomes almost unbearable or you have a noticeable loss of function. Fortunately, recent advances in arthroscopic surgery make this a safer and more effective option than it was a few years ago.

There are a wide range of surgical procedures. The most extreme includes removing portions of the vertebrae *(laminectomy)* and inserting either bone chips or metallic devices to cause the bones above and below the surgery site to fuse together. This surgery requires the patient to spend several days in the hospital and is followed by a recovery period that often includes a physical therapy program. On the other end of the surgical spectrum, there is *microdiscectomy*, a relatively simple outpatient procedure that removes just a small portion of a disc. The correct surgical approach is determined by the size and location of the herniation, or the degree of degeneration. Finding the right surgeon—one who will take the time to discuss all options and alternatives, and one who has a solid reputation for performing these procedures—is important to your outcome.

Intradiscal Electrothermal Therapy

In *intradiscal electrothermal therapy* (IDET), a thin wire is inserted into the bulging or protruding disc that is thought to be producing back pain. An electrical current is then run through the wire, causing it to heat up and shrink the disc. To date, the procedure has not proven to be effective, and patient satisfaction studies have not been favorable (Davis et al. 2004). In the 1980s, a similar attempt to reduce the size of bulging discs with chemical injections (*chemonucleolysis*) yielded less than satisfactory results, and the procedure is no longer utilized.

Radio Lesioning

Radio lesioning is employed when the suspected cause of pain is nerve root irritation within the joint. Pulsed radio frequencies are used to obliterate the nerves, thereby relieving the pain. Although radio lesioning can be an effective pain reliever, the relief is usually temporary, and in most cases the procedure needs to be repeated every six months to one year. The overall benefit of radio lesioning remains unproven (Niemisto et al. 2003).

Trigger Point Injections

Trigger point injections are local anesthetic injections administered directly into sites of severe muscle pain and spasm that have not responded to other therapies. The hope is that when the affected area is numbed, the pain will subside and the spasm will decrease. Trigger point injections provide only temporary relief and have received mixed reviews. Trigger point injections should not be done at multiple sites.

Think Back

The wide range of available conservative treatments—from physical therapy and chiropractic to acupuncture and yoga—can be helpful in treating up to 95 percent of all cases of chronic neck and back pain. Most therapies have about the same rate of success, and the key to finding the right therapy is in finding the right therapist. Choose a therapist who's willing to engage in an open dialogue that focuses on you and not the treatment. The 15-50 rule is the best way to assess the value of the therapy.

If your pain has not responded to conservative treatments and you've had more than four weeks of severe and unremitting pain that is causing loss of function in an arm or leg, aggressive or invasive treatments such as injections or surgeries may be necessary. These treatments carry more risks and side effects than conservative therapies, so choosing the right doctor is just as important as choosing the right treatment. When you have to consider aggressive therapies, start with the least invasive of the appropriate procedures, either medications or injections. If they are not helpful, you may need to consider surgery. Surgical procedures are improving daily, and you should investigate your options with a surgeon who is open to your questions and cares about your concerns.

Even with the right treatments in place, you are still going to need the right frame of mind to motivate yourself to see things through. The success of self-directed home care, conservative therapies, and aggressive treatments all depend upon your commitment and desire to optimize your results. Chapter 8 will provide the motivation, reassurance, and additional supportive recommendations to help you stop the recurrence of chronic neck and back pain.

CHAPTER 8

Overcoming Chronic Pain

Every treatment plan from a physician, physical therapist, chiropractor, or acupuncturist begins with a diagnosis and ends with the treatment goals. And until recently, regardless of the diagnosis, the most common treatment goals were relief of pain, increased function, and increased strength. However, with recognition of the fact that an unnecessarily large percentage of acute pain cases become chronic (Reeser et al. 2001), the main goal of all neck and back treatment plans should be to escape the traps that lead to chronic pain. Unfortunately, if you are reading this book, you have probably already developed chronic pain, and you might think that it's too late for you to escape those traps. Well, it's not. Overcoming chronic pain and avoiding the traps that lead to chronic pain are one and the same.

MAKING A COMMITMENT

There are two paths pain takes to become chronic: the psychological path discussed in chapter 3, and the physical paths discussed in chapters 4 and 5. If you are going to avoid chronic pain or escape the chronic pain you're in, then you'd better know how to avoid the traps that can draw you down. The first and most important step is to get at the physical cause of your problem as quickly as possible. This is called *early intervention,* and it has been proven to significantly reduce the fears, suffering, and costs that come with chronic pain (Gatchel et al. 2003; Wand et al. 2004). But in cases where early intervention is no longer an option, the next best thing you can do—even before starting a treatment program—is to make a wholehearted commitment to stick to whichever treatment approach you ultimately choose.

Relieving symptoms is the easy part of treating back pain, and almost anything you do will be helpful in that regard. However, reversing the tissue changes that have been there for years takes uncommon resolve. Only patients who *choose* to be rid of chronic pain succeed at this. Your muscles and joints work hard every day, and they need stimulation, stretching, and motion every day as well. Therefore, you must take a vow that no matter how hard it is or how long you have to stay with it, you will never give up until you are completely satisfied with the effort you've put in and the results you have achieved. This doesn't mean you'll have to go for months of formal treatment in therapy offices. It means you will have to make a daily commitment to rebuild the pain-free back you deserve.

Prolonged pain and tightness cause tissues to change in size, shape, consistency, strength, and flexibility, and a month or two of therapy will never achieve the lasting changes necessary to prevent the reoccurrences that lead to chronic pain. Given that it has likely taken years for you to develop aberrant tissue patterns, you must accept the fact that it will take months of dedicated and conscientious work to begin reversing those changes. It is illogical and implausible to expect that you can undo years of strain and neglect by going to a physical therapist or chiropractor three times a week for six or eight weeks. Even the best therapy or advice in the world will never make up for a lack of dedication and the necessary follow-through.

In the great majority of cases, there is absolutely no reason neck and back pain sufferers cannot jump the same daunting hurdles that sufferers of other debilitating conditions have overcome in their lives. I don't mean to minimize the pain you have endured or the struggles you have been through.

You have every right to feel bitter, discouraged, frustrated, and perhaps improperly cared for by those you have consulted in the past. But if teenage amputees are able to bear the loss of a leg, strap on a prosthetic limb, and then train rigorously to run high school track, play college football, or learn how to downhill ski, then you can find the desire, strength, and determination to make great strides, too. If special-needs children are able to muster the mettle and compete in Special Olympics with the fervor, effervescence, and joy that can uplift the spirits of an entire stadium, then you can find the courage and fortitude to compete with yourself to improve your outcome as well. If your determination and commitment are ongoing and unwavering, then how can your results be anything less than spectacular? Even if you feel that you've put in your fair share of time with doctors and therapists over the years, you may have to come to terms with the possibility that you haven't even scratched the surface of what you can and must do. There is no therapy, treatment, exercise, surgery, or pill more powerful or longer lasting than your tireless effort to succeed.

Ask people who suffer from ongoing or periodic lower back pain about their commitment to staying pain free, and I guarantee you will receive a less-than-inspired response. They'll likely tell you about what they should be doing or make an excuse for not putting in the necessary efforts. Yet, ask people who are no longer shackled by periodic flare-ups how they have conquered their pain, and a smile will surely come to their face as they begin telling you how they've done it. It takes a certain attitude to achieve this level of engagement, and that attitude comes from a strong understanding that the goal is real and possible. Where there is little understanding, there is little hope and only a faint likelihood you'll follow through.

The key to accomplishing this goal, to conceiving of and then achieving a pain-free neck and back, is to move away from fear and negative expectations. Through the first seven chapters, you've been given the practical information and scientific basis for living pain free. But, if your deepest expectations are pessimistic, then you have to change those, too. Knowing that a pain-free back is a real possibility is the first vital change you must make. With this understanding, all the additional necessary steps are easily undertaken. Without the understanding that a pain-free back is possible, you will wind up fighting yourself every step of the way.

In its innate ability to repair and renew itself, your body is far more intelligent and dynamic than your scientific mind. Yet most people have intellectualized themselves into favoring their shortcomings and weaknesses above their body's strengths and nature's truest tendencies. Consequently, it is easy for them to believe there is nothing that can be done for chronic neck and back pain, so nothing is exactly what they do. They continually repeat the same mistakes that contributed to their pain in the first place.

In the simplest form, your neck and back are nothing more than flesh and bone. They grow, they change, they adapt, they scar, they heal, and like all flesh and bone they give you life. And in return, what you give to them determines how they grow, how they change, how they adapt, how they scar, and most importantly how they heal. In essence, what you do for your neck and back will ultimately influence the quality of life they give you. Now, is a few minutes a day of simple home stretching and exercise too much to ask? If millions of other people just like you can do this, so can you.

SELF-INVESTIGATION

Self-investigation, or looking at your entire lifestyle for clues as to why you might be in pain, is an extremely valuable and necessary tool in ending chronic pain. Very few doctors or therapists will take the time to sit down with you and go through an hour-by-hour examination of what you do and how it affects your spine, but if you don't go through that process, there is a good chance you are missing something very simple that is hindering your progress. The poor results seen in many chronic neck and back pain cases can be a manifestation of things people are either doing to themselves or not doing for themselves. An investigation of how you may be inadvertently contributing to the problem is a great place to begin looking for clues as to why you developed this pain and why it is not going away. Here are two examples that illustrate the importance of self-investigation.

In the first case, I was treating a young woman who developed chronic neck pain over a two-year period that various therapies failed to relieve. There was no history of trauma or injury, and as far as she could remember, the pain simply started one morning when she woke up with a stiff neck. After two weeks of treatment, even though she diligently performed the stretching and range of motion exercises, she said the stiffness was only slightly improved. This woman was employed as a retail clerk, and I questioned her carefully about the job requirements and her normal daily activities. We didn't uncover any obvious heavy lifting or prolonged positioning tasks that could account for her continued pain and minimal response to treatment. She was unhappy, and I was confused.

Lightning finally struck in the third week. I happened to walk into the waiting room and noticed her sitting with a cell phone between her shoulder and ear while she was getting something out of her bag. When she came into the examination room, I asked her if she spent much time in that position. She explained that she didn't, really, because the cell phone was too thin and it hurt too much. So I asked her if she spent much time on the phone at home, and she said no, not too much time. So then I asked how much time was "not too much." Well, by now you may have guessed the problem. When she said she spent "only two to three hours a night" with her head in that tilted position, I almost fell over. Here she was trying to do everything possible to treat and correct her problem, while without ever giving it a second thought, and as part of her regular evening routine, she was doing something that had probably caused her pain and was certainly prolonging it. Now although this may seem like an obvious and extreme example to you, this very evening, millions of neck pain sufferers are going to either spend several hours holding a phone between their ear and shoulder or fall asleep on the couch with their head and neck bolstered to one side by three or four pillows.

The next example is a well-educated, athletic, and six-foot-tall middle-aged man who spent most of every evening on a charming 1940s-style five-foot-long couch. Although he vigorously exercised three times a week for the general health benefits, at night he would lie on his back watching TV with his head propped up on one arm of the couch and both legs extended straight out over the other arm. He stayed in his human V position for several hours, yet he could never figure out why he woke in pain every morning. There he was, thinking he was doing everything right to stay in shape, without ever realizing he was causing his own problem by the "shape" he was staying in.

Investigating the source of your pain may take you right to the core of what you most love to do. By now I hope you know how important daily exercise is, but ironically, there is only one thing harder than getting people to start exercising, and that is trying to get avid or extreme exercisers to slow down. A three-times-a-week singles tennis player would rather endure chronic neck and upper back pain from serves and overheads before ever considering playing doubles once a week. Most golfers would do anything to take a few strokes off their game, but ask them to not play for two weeks and you'll see grown men and women start to beg like children. But the most passionate of all physical exercise enthusiasts are the self-proclaimed gym and road rats. These are the people who believe that without extensive exercise, they will suddenly shrink into oblivion, or that their exercise "high" is the mandatory spiritual equivalent of daily prayer. Getting them to stop or slow down is almost impossible. Repetitive stress and strain can contribute to chronic pain, and they can come from anything you do regularly, exercise included. Too much of a good thing is no longer a good thing when it causes or prolongs your pain.

Finally, every self-investigation must include a good hard look at the leading cause of self-induced pain: prolonged positioning or repetitive movements at work. It doesn't matter whether you are a data entry clerk, steam pipe fitter, scientist, or dentist; spend enough time in one position or constantly perform the same movements, and you will pay the price of chronic pain. Going in to work tomorrow and demanding a new high-back leather chair or expecting the factory to reconfigure an assembly line to fit your needs is obviously not the answer. But if you believe your work is contributing to your pain, then you must devise different ways to do that work. Some tips and suggestions are provided later in this chapter. The one thing you cannot do is keep repeating the same pain-producing routines and expect to achieve different results. That will never happen.

What your entire self-investigation will ultimately come down to is limiting or removing the detrimental habits and initiating or maximizing the beneficial ones. A great way to begin your own self-investigation is to make a chart of what you do on an hourly basis. You can then assign a number from 1 to 5 to each activity based on how significantly you feel it contributes to your pain. This can be a very eye-opening experience, giving you valuable clues about how you can alter your activities to reduce your pain.

Time of day	Activity	Position	Location and degree of pain	Correction
11:00 P.M.— 7:00 A.M.	sleeping	on stomach	lower back, 4	sleep on side
7:00 A.M.— 7:30 A.M.	drive to work	sitting in car	lower back, 3	try lumbar pillow
8:00 A.M.— noon	work as a rodeo cowboy	flying through the air	neck and lower back, 5	find a new job
noon— 1:00 P.M.	lunch	walking around	lower back, 1	do more walking
1:00 P.M.— 2:00 P.M.	watch video of morning ride	sitting	neck pain, 2	move neck more

Figure 8.1: Sample Self-Investigation Chart

Self-Investigation Chart

Time of day	Activity	Position	Location and degree of pain	Correction

I know that going through this process may seem a little silly, but writing this information down will help you uncover hidden contributing factors and also remind you what you should and should not be doing. Once you have completed a thorough self-investigation, the next step is to begin taking the daily measures that will counter these factors. This is the beginning of good spinal hygiene.

SPINAL HYGIENE

You know the difference between good and poor dental hygiene, and you know how those differences affect your teeth and gums. What you may not have realized is that the differences between good and poor spinal hygiene have the same kind of effect on your spine, muscles, and bones.

Exercise

The single most important task of good dental hygiene is regular brushing. It removes waste from around the teeth and stimulates blood flow to the gums. The single most important task of good spinal hygiene is regular exercise, which removes waste from within the muscles and stimulates the functions of muscles, joints, and bones. For your neck and back, exercise is the fountain of youth. It keeps the muscles flexible, the joints loose, and the bones strong.

Regardless of what you may have heard, it doesn't really matter what exercise you do, as long as you get some movement and stimulation into your spine. If you have been sedentary for a while, a modest walking program—perhaps a ten- to fifteen-minute daily stroll—is a great place to start. Each week, try to extend your time by a few minutes, until you can comfortably walk thirty minutes without stopping. The goal is to effectively exercise your spine without stressing yourself physically or mentally. I recommend you go about it in a relaxed manner. If you eventually feel like picking up the pace, it should help your cardiovascular system, but the faster rate will make no difference to your spine.

The major reason people stop exercising is boredom, so it is a good idea to select two or three different routes for your walk. Anything you can do to help change the program will help keep your interest. If you are like most people, once you start enjoying the benefits of exercising, you'll actually look forward to doing it. Other great exercises for your spine include swimming, dancing, moderate jogging, tai chi, yoga, or Pilates. All of these routines are excellent daily activities to help avoid chronic pain and maintain good spinal health. Although they do not take the place of the directed stretching or range of motion exercises, they are beneficial supplements.

Posture and Positioning

After exercise, posture and positioning are the other important factors you must pay attention to. They play a vital role in everything you do, including standing, sitting, sleeping, and lifting. Your spine is designed around three basic curves that maximize the mechanical advantages for weight bearing and distribution. These curves act like arches in bridge construction, transferring the loads and distributing the stress very efficiently. Looking at your spine from the side, there is a slight forward curve in your neck, a larger backward curve to the middle of your spine, and a second forward curve in the lower back. And while it's normal for the degree or size of these curves to vary from person to person, you should try to maintain good posture whenever possible.

If viewed from the side, in a good standing or sitting posture, the center of your head, the middle of your shoulders, and the center of your hips are in one straight line. This position reinforces the three spinal curves and reduces the structural strain on the muscles, joints, ligaments, and discs. The best way to achieve this position is by elevating your shoulders upward and backward directly over your hips, then raising your

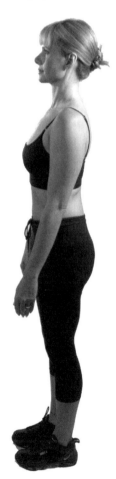

Figure 8.2: Standing Posture

chin slightly so you are looking straight ahead. This is the same neutral position that was referred to in the exercises in chapter 6.

Maintaining good posture is especially important when you are going to be in the same position for a long period of time. While frequent changes of position allow the downward force of your body weight to be shifted, stationary positions cause the downward force of your body weight to remain constantly focused in one direction. This results in a buildup of weight-bearing stress and strain on the affected tissues. Maintaining the three spinal curves helps the body automatically and efficiently transfer the weight-bearing loads, thereby relieving much of the mechanical strain on the muscles, joints, and discs. Because prolonged standing and sitting is sometimes unavoidable, here are some simple tips that may help.

PROPER STANDING POSTURE

One of the most common complaints I hear from people with lower back pain is that they get increased pain when they have to stand in one place. This occurs because the transfer of weight-bearing loads is not taking place, and a physical strain is allowed to build up. If you find yourself in this predicament and cannot move around to change your position, you are going to have to change your weight distribution by changing your stance. The best way to do this is to frequently shift your weight back and forth from one leg to the other. If possible, prop one foot up on a small box or step, and occasionally alternate feet. Western tavern and saloon owners took advantage of this simple weight-transferring concept and devised the brass bar foot rail. This invention kept their customers comfortable enough to continue standing and drinking at the bar long enough to drink themselves into a reclining position.

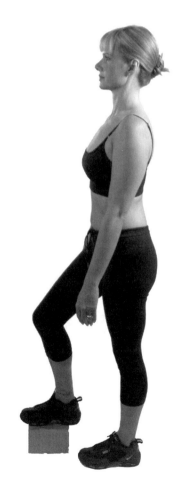

Figure 8.3: Standing with One Foot on a Box

Even if you find yourself having to belly up to the kitchen sink instead of a bar, you can still use the same weight transfer trick by opening one of the undersink cabinet doors, propping one foot up on the cabinet floor, and occasionally switching feet. Not only will this help transfer your weight, it will give you additional forward-bending leverage while you are leaning into the sink. Cashiers or factory line workers can also take advantage of this tip by placing a small box under their workstation and using it in the exact same manner. The most important thing to do when you're on your feet and cannot move around is to keep changing the weight bearing from one leg to the other.

PROPER SITTING POSTURE

Many people with back pain have jobs that require prolonged sitting. In most cases, these people are leaning or hunching forward over a desk, causing the curve in the lower back to straighten or reverse. Now, instead of the lower back transferring weight loads to the hips and into the seat, the lower back becomes the focal point of the load, and the strain builds relentlessly.

There is only one stable sitting posture for the lower back, and this is with a forward lumbar curve.

If you spend significant time in a sitting position, then you have to either remember to keep the arch in your back or get a small pillow or lumbar cushion to keep it there for you. On long car or plane rides, it's best to place a small pillow or folded-up face towel in the small of your back, just above the waistline. This will help keep the forward arch in your back. Large lumbar cushions or internal lumbar supports in car seats don't fit everyone perfectly, and they are difficult or impossible to adjust. A small cushion works best because you can occasionally move it up or

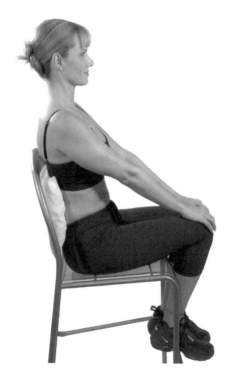

Figure 8.4: Sitting with a Lumbar Pillow

down and side to side to keep changing your position. Of course, the best thing you can do for prolonged sitting is to get up and move around. You will be greatly surprised how beneficial it can be to take two ten-second laps around your desk every half hour. Those twenty seconds of walking will more than make up for the loss of concentration and work productivity caused by the increased pain and stiffness that come from not walking. When it comes to either prolonged standing or prolonged sitting, remember to transfer your weight from side to side, and keep the arch in your lower back.

PROLONGED NECK POSITIONING

A third common complaint relates to neck pain caused by prolonged positioning, most often from using the computer or reading in bed. And while switching the weight in your legs and keeping the arch in your lower back are the easiest ways to deflect the mechanical lower back stress of prolonged positioning, the best way to deflect neck stress is through regular movement that won't require a change in your entire body position. Whenever your head and neck are going to be in one position for extended periods, it is essential to perform the gentle range of motion exercises two to three times an hour. (See chapter 6 for review of the exercises.) If you know you are going to be at your workstation or reading in bed for a long time, every twenty to thirty minutes, you should stop and move your neck. The entire cycle of five repetitions in each direction will take less than a minute, and if you do the exercises regularly, they will probably prevent much of the tightness and uncomfortable stiffness of prolonged positioning from ever developing in the first place.

PROPER SLEEPING POSITIONS

The fourth major complaint is from patients who frequently wake up in the morning with neck or lower back pain. The question they ask is, "What is the best position for sleeping?" If you have acute neck pain, you want to lie flat on your back with your shoulders and neck slightly elevated. This will usually take two pillows, one placed at the top of the shoulders and a second thicker pillow to support your head and neck.

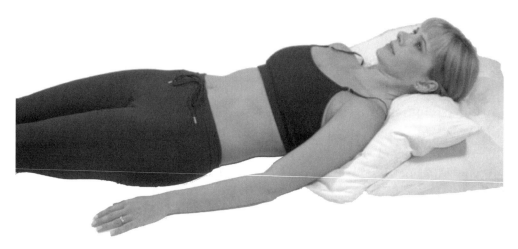

Figure 8.5: Pillow Placement for Acute Neck Pain

When you have acute lower back pain, you must find a position that relieves the pain and at the same time supports the lower back. A commonly recommended position is lying flat on your back with a thin pillow under your neck and a thick pillow under your knees.

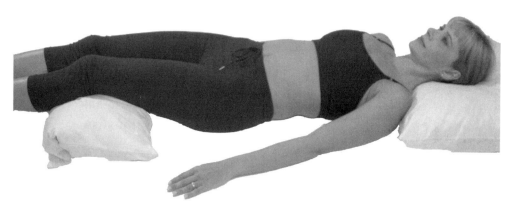

Figure 8.6: Lying on Back with Pillow Under Knees

This position is supposed to take pressure off the lower back, and although it is comfortable for brief periods, because the full pressure of your body weight is bearing straight down on your back, you may find it difficult to stay in this position for an entire night's sleep. By rolling partway to the side (the side opposite the pain, if one side of your back hurts worse) and placing a thick, long body pillow behind your spine, you can relieve the pressure and support your lower back at the same time. This position should allow you to get a much more comfortable night's sleep.

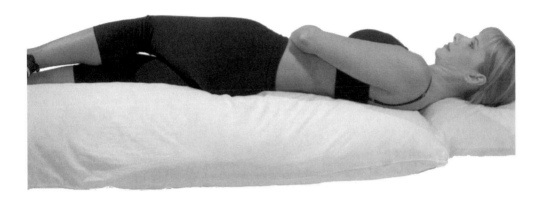

Figure 8.7: Lying on Side with Pillow Behind Spine

When there is no acute neck or back pain, you can sleep in almost any comfortable position. However, if you regularly go to sleep feeling fine and then wake up with pain or stiffness, you probably sleep on your stomach, and that habit has to be changed. When you are on your stomach, the lumbar spine is completely unsupported, and the neck is forced to turn to one side. This causes a prolonged strain on the spinal tendons and ligaments and leaves you feeling like you've just slept on a log instead of like a log. If you have a hard time breaking the stomach-sleeping habit, try lying on one side with the top leg slightly bent at the knee, and then place an extra-long, thick pillow under your chest. This will give you the same feeling as sleeping on your stomach, but most of the unsupported downward strain will now be taken away from the lower back. Some people have found that placing a small pillow under the top knee or between the knees also helps relieve lower back strain.

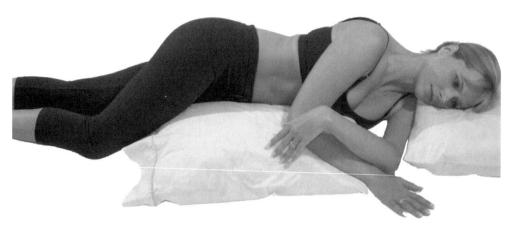

Figure 8.8a: Pillow Under Chest

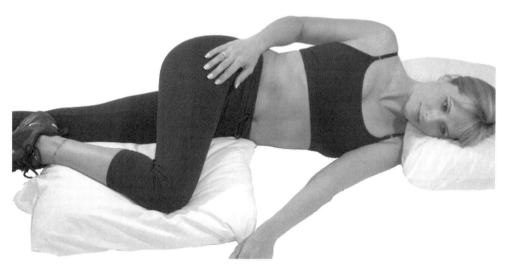

Figure 8.8b: Lying on Side with Pillow Under One Knee

It is also essential to properly support your neck at night. The key to relieving neck strain is to make sure your head, neck, and spine all remain in a straight line parallel to the plane of the bed. If you prefer sleeping on your back, use any regular-sized pillow that is comfortable and to your liking. It is important to get your entire neck onto and supported by the pillow. If your pillow is only supporting the back of your head, if it is too thick, or if you are using two pillows, your head and chin are probably being pushed forward, straining the tendons and ligaments of your neck. If your pillow is too thin, chances are the forward curve in your neck is not getting any support, and this will also result in unnecessary strain.

When you sleep on your side, the best way to support your head and neck is by taking a fairly thick but soft pillow, bunching it up, and then tucking it under your neck and head. Too thick a pillow will push your head to one side, and too thin a pillow will allow your head and neck to sway downward.

You can buy contoured pillows designed to position your neck, but they don't fit everyone exactly right, and they cannot be manipulated as you change positions. Any modestly thick and soft pillow that can conform to your preferred sleeping position will provide more than adequate and comfortable support.

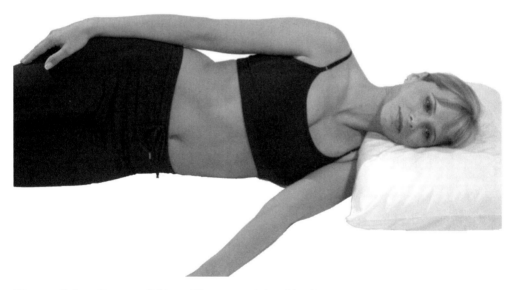

Figure 8.9a: Proper Pillow Placement for Neck

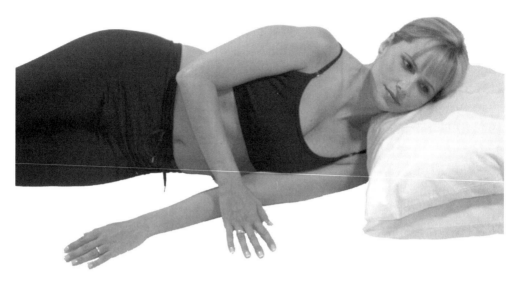

Figure 8.9b: Pillow Too Thick for Neck

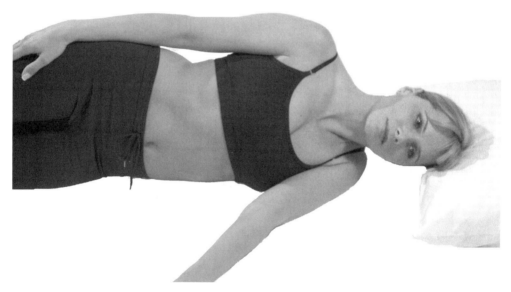

Figure 8.9c: Pillow Too Thin for Neck

There Will Be Setbacks

After you have done everything you should do (targeted massage, range of motion exercises, directed stretching, self-investigation, and spinal hygiene) there is one last thing to remember. There will be setbacks. Only a handful of people ever go from constant or frequent episodes of pain to absolutely no pain ever again. But don't get discouraged. The longer you stay committed to your program of stretching, exercise, and massage the less likely it is that those setbacks will occur and the less severe they should be. I bring this to your attention because if and when a flare-up does occur you must be ready to meet it head on. It won't do you any good to say things like "Here I go again," or "I must be back to square one." Those things aren't true. If you've been diligent about keeping up with the stretching and exercises then even though you may feel like it's that same old pain, it actually isn't. Your neck and back have made some significant changes that should make these flare-ups mere shells of what they were. And although your initial interpretation is "Here I go again," the reality usually amounts to something much less than that. Because your spine is in better condition from all the hard work you have put in, the typical week or two of pain that flare-ups once caused could now be limited to not much more than a day or two.

When a flare-up does occur don't get discouraged because that will only work against you. Your back didn't "go out" so there is no reason to "freak out" or "fear out." You are going to treat a flare-up as if it were simple acute neck or back pain. Depending on the symptoms and recommendations discussed in earlier chapters, you will apply ice, heat, medication, rest, or exercise, as warranted. And after you have gotten over one or two of these flare-ups, you will come to realize just how magnificent your spine is and just how wonderfully it seeks to restore itself. As time goes by the frequency of flare-ups will diminish, their intensity will abate, and you'll trust in your spine to respond with all its miraculous recuperative powers.

Think Back

Overcoming chronic pain and avoiding chronic pain are one and the same. Try to get to the physical cause of your problem as soon as possible, and once you have chosen a program to treat the physical aspects, make a wholehearted commitment to see that plan through. This takes dedication and motivation; you must not quit until you are pain free. Because chronic pain is often reinforced by something you are either doing or not doing, an investigation into your daily activities will give you vital clues about how you can avoid and overcome many of the factors that are causing or contributing to your pain. The self-investigation must be followed by a plan for good spinal hygiene that includes proper posture and standing, sitting, and sleeping positions.

CHAPTER 9

Success Stories

My years in practice have been filled with personal and professional achievements, the most rewarding of which have been helping some wonderful patients regain their health. It is through the extraordinary willingness of these people to share their successes and their failures, their triumphs, and their hardships that I have come to appreciate the awesome power of the doctor-patient relationship. At its highest level, this is an unrestricted two-way street with both lanes converging for the benefit of the patient. The word "doctor" comes from a Latin word meaning to teach, educate, or draw forth. Doctors who limit their practice to diagnosing ailments and prescribing treatments miss out on the great opportunity, responsibility, and joy of educating patients and inspiring their capacity for health and well-being. The word "patient" comes from a Latin word meaning to endure, to persist, or to outlast. With that comes an implicit obligation to not give up, to hang in there, and to try anything and everything possible to persevere and succeed. When doctors do everything they can to educate and draw forth patients whose desire is to persevere and thrive, the chances of a successful result become greatly enhanced. Not only does the patient benefit from this relationship, but the doctor also takes away a little something that can be used to assist other patients. Here are a few experiences that helped change the way I treat and see patients and how they see themselves.

■ "You're the Doctor?"

When I first opened my office twenty-five years ago, I certainly didn't know everything there was to know about neck and back pain, and like every other first-year practitioner I was young, inexperienced, and probably a little naive. However, I did know that I was about to embark on an important journey, gaining valuable knowledge from the kind of practical insight and experience no laboratory or textbook could ever provide. I also knew that the key to processing this information would come from open-minded observation and the flexibility to put new ideas to work. If I could just listen carefully enough, or just watch long enough, then surely somewhere down the road I would be a better doctor than I was on day one.

My very first patient was a forty-five-year-old well-dressed and well-groomed accountant who expected quality service and a high level of knowledge from those around him. Looking back on it now, I can only imagine the combination of fear and disappointment he must have felt when I first walked into the examination room. He was probably expecting to see a figure of equal professional stature, and instead in walks a skinny twenty-six-year-old swimming in a lab coat two sizes too big. He looked up, and with all the politeness and decorum he could muster, he asked in a disbelieving tone, "You're the doctor?" Hoping my insecurity wasn't overly obvious, I briefly glanced around the room to make sure he was talking to me. Unfortunately he was, and the only response I could manage was to jokingly retort in my own disbelieving tone, "You're the patient?" Luckily he had a sense of humor, and we got along just fine. But without ever knowing it, this man had thrown down the gauntlet, and the challenge to be "The Doctor" has been mine ever since. Some things have changed since then—I no longer wear a lab coat, I'm not quite as skinny, and those early insecurities are long gone. But the challenge to listen, to educate, to draw forth, and to strive for the benefit of the patient has always remained.

■ "Dat's da Shpot"

When I graduated school, I was well-trained in diagnosis, physical examination, and the art of spinal manipulation. There wasn't a bone in the spine I couldn't confidently move, and there wasn't a neck or back problem I thought I couldn't diagnose or properly treat. In some cases, that may have meant referring the patient to someone else, but at least I knew what to treat and what not to treat, when to refer and when not to. It was 1979, and most patients who were seeing chiropractors had first gone to medical doctors with-out much success. They wanted something better than the temporary relief of medications and heating pads, and SMT was the only new alternative. Chiropractic and SMT were losing their undeserved mystical and maligned reputation. With this new approach, patients were improving beyond what they had previously experienced with other therapies.

But what about the patients for whom spinal manipulation was either inappropriate or ineffective? The only alternatives were physical therapy and treatments that had already failed many patients before they ever came to see me. I was resigned to the idea that if SMT wasn't going to help them, neither was I. All of that was about to change when I got my first and possibly most important lesson in listening to the patient.

In 1983, my reception room had a large picture window that looked out onto a tree-lined two-lane road, and if you happened to peer out any morning at 10:45, chances were you would see a tall, very thin, striking figure: a finely dressed older lady in matching patent leather pumps quick-stepping herself into town. She made her way with an unusual determination in her stride, eyes and head fixed straight down. I remember commenting to my receptionist that this woman would probably walk right into traffic one day because all she ever saw was one foot moving in front of the other. But to her credit, even in the coldest weather, there she was in her woolen winter whites, making her daily trek back and forth from town.

One morning at 10:45, my receptionist came running into my office and said, "Guess who just came in? It's her, Mrs.—you know, the walker." After the timid woman (whom I shall refer to as Mrs. Walker) repeatedly apologized for not having an appointment, she filled out the initial paperwork, and I began taking her case history. She complained of left-sided upper back pain which began six months earlier and occasionally radiated into her left shoul-der and arm. A friend of hers referred her to my office, but at that time she was afraid to come in. She continued to try several home remedies, including ice and heat, but nothing seemed to help.

I assumed the fears that originally kept Mrs. Walker away from my office were from not knowing what to expect or from common misconceptions about chiropractic. I was accustomed to those kinds of patient fears, and overall, there didn't seem to be anything unusual about Mrs. Walker's case. Then, I casually asked her, "Why, after passing here every day for the past six months, did you finally decide to come in now?" Her eyes welled up with water and her lips began to quiver. Through a very thick accent, in the very softest of voices,

Mrs. Walker began to tell me about her life in Germany during the late 1930s and early 1940s. As a young woman, she witnessed terrible atrocities and was unable to offer any help. Her fear was not of chiropractic or of spinal manipulation. She was afraid that because of my heritage, I would associate her with those atrocities and not be willing to treat her. Obviously that wasn't the case, and after I was able to saddle my own emotions, I proceeded to look for the physical cause of Mrs. Walker's problem.

There she was, eighty-four years old, thin as a rail, fragile, as breakable as an egg, and in significant pain. Spinal manipulation would not have been appropriate, and there weren't a lot of other therapeutic options that offered much hope. Yet somehow I found myself drawn to this case in a way that I had not been to any other. I had to do something for this patient. On her second visit, as I was applying some very light and general massage to her upper back, Mrs. Walker cried out faintly but emphatically, "Dat's da shpot." It took me a few seconds to absorb what she was saying, and after I figured out what "Dat's da shpot" meant, I decided to continue working on that location. We repeated the procedure over the next few visits, and Mrs. Walker began to improve with each treatment.

This was not the discovery of targeted massage, but my observation of what it was able to accomplish for Mrs. Walker led me to start applying it to other patients as well. As time went on and the successes with targeted massage continued, a new office anthem was created. "Dat's da shpot" became the battle cry for those in need of relief from muscular neck and back pain. Skeptics will likely point out that Mrs. Walker's case may have had significant psychological overlay that could account for her results, and they may be right. What Mrs. Walker's case cannot account for are the similar results seen in those patients without such psychological overlay. After all, truck drivers, construction workers, and teenagers weren't exactly pouring their emotionally tender hearts out to me as I was digging away at the spasm in their back. Mrs. Walker's case is only interesting and important for two reasons. First, it was my initial experience with targeted massage; and secondly, there was one person whom Mrs. Walker finally did help. And although I never had the opportunity to tell her, in some way her legacy lives on and will hopefully bring help to thousands of other people. Targeted massage has become a therapeutic success story in its own right. Mrs. Walker's case just happened to be my first success at it.

■ "Your Aunt Is on the Phone"

Several years ago, I was sitting on the back deck when my wife came out and handed me the phone, saying, "It's your aunt from Texas." After we spoke for a few minutes, my aunt started telling me about a problem she was having with her neck and upper back. She was feeling excessive stiffness and tightness, hearing grinding noises, and experiencing a general ache. She also mentioned that she was occasionally waking up in the middle of the night with tingling in her arms and hands that quickly faded if she changed her position. Years earlier when I was visiting, she'd had a similar condition, which had responded quickly to some spinal manipulation. This time I was 1,500 miles away, she had already tried some less-than-effective manipulation, and she was now seeing a physical therapist who had her exercising as if she were training for the Olympic weight lifting team.

Every doctor knows that diagnosing and treating patients over the phone is an ethically gray area. But when your aunt from Texas calls, you have no choice—it's time to "cowboy up." She was in desperate need of relief, and I had to suggest something other than what had already failed. Anything that required hands-on treatment was impractical, so the only option left was for her to stop the strength training and begin some directed range of motion exercises. Although I had been recommending these exercises for some time, I always prescribed them in combination with manipulation and massage. Prior to my aunt's call, I had never relied on directed range of motion as an isolated therapy, and I was unaware of their stand-alone potential.

We spent some time going over the exercises, and I explained the importance of doing them on a regular basis. When I called her a few days later, her complaints were still there, but she had already noticed improvement in the movement and less overall stiffness. The enthusiasm in her voice made me feel almost as relieved as she was. She continued with the exercises until her symptoms were completely gone, and to this day she does them several times a week. Even in the absence of any other therapies, directed range of motion can be a powerful therapeutic instrument.

■ There's Nothing Like a Vacation

The next opportunity to use directed range of motion as an isolated therapy presented itself in a fairly unusual way. A sixty-five-year-old gentleman scheduled his initial appointment in my office just days before he was leaving on a six-week European vacation. Like my aunt, he had neck pain and stiffness, only his had been there for several years, along with an almost constant numbness and tingling in his hands. He had already seen an orthopedist and a neurologist, and their testing confirmed he had nerve damage from herniated discs and degenerative joint disease. I explained to this gentleman that the last thing I wanted to do was upset the applecart just before he left on a six-week vacation. His condition had been there for quite some time, and I wanted to wait until he got back before starting any procedures. He agreed, but then asked if there was anything he could do while he was away to start the ball rolling and help relieve a little of the stiffness. Almost reluctantly, I suggested he try the gentle directed range of motion exercises on a very limited basis.

Seven weeks later, a relaxed, well-tanned gentleman sat in my examination room with a very interesting story to tell. Yes, the castles of Spain were inspiring, but what had really amazed him was how much better his neck had become. After spending six weeks conscientiously sipping wines, faithfully basking in the Spanish sun, and religiously working on his range of motion exercises, he could now report a significant improvement in his symptoms. And by his own admission, the sun and the wine contributed very little to the positive physical changes. I asked how he was so sure that it wasn't the combination of the exercises and his restful vacation lifestyle, and he responded that he had been retired for several years and his lifestyle was essentially the same regardless of which continent he was on. That kind of response was good enough for me. He was certain the range of motion exercises had significantly increased his movement and decreased his pain, and it also accounted for another unexpected benefit. The numbness and tingling in his right hand was 50 percent better, and it had almost completely disappeared from his left hand.

This success story not only confirmed the effectiveness of directed range of motion for pain and stiffness, it opened up an entirely new application. Directed range of motion exercises could help with the neurological symptoms of numbness and tingling in the extremities that are associated with herniated discs and degenerative joint disease. And now that Mr. Vacation was going to be back in town for a while, I couldn't wait to see what would happen when spinal manipulation, deep massage, and directed stretching were added into the mix. Luckily, I had learned that it is always better to be cautiously optimistic than it is to make bold or grandiose predictions. In this case, the additional therapies gave him only limited additional improvement, but they never had anywhere near the substantial benefit that the directed range of motion exercises did. Neither Mr. Vacation nor I were disappointed, however. He was more than happy to be rid of the chronic neck pain and stiffness along with a good percentage of the numbness and tingling in his hands. I was excited to have seen further confirmation of the benefits that directed range of motion can offer.

■ A Concert of Therapies

This next case illustrates the effectiveness of combining all the directed therapies. An eighty-two-year-old man entered my office complaining of chronic lower back pain. During the previous two weeks the pain had progressed, and it was now traveling from his buttock into his left leg and foot. This was an energetic man, still busy selling real estate and playing golf twice a week. He had to travel forty miles round-trip to my office, and he had no patience for the pain that was interfering with his active lifestyle. He had *scoliosis* (curvature) of the lower back so significant that his pant legs had to be altered to different lengths to account for the left hip being almost two full inches higher than the right. He believed the scoliosis was responsible for his chronic lower back pain, and he had learned to curtail his activities when the pain got too bad. But now that the pain was almost constant and traveling into his leg, he was looking for something effective and noninvasive to relieve the condition. He knew the scoliosis had been there for his entire life and did not expect anything to change that; he just wanted the pain to go away.

After three office visits that included targeted massage, gentle and low-force spinal manipulation techniques, and detailed instruction in directed stretching and range of motion exercises, this man had made an almost 100 percent recovery. The chronic lower back pain was reduced to a mild, intermittent soreness, and the buttock and leg pain were completely gone.

I don't know if any one of the three procedures was more responsible for his improvement than the others, and in this particular case, I really didn't care. There was no reason not to apply all three procedures as early as possible in the treatment, and that is exactly what we did. This was not a random "try every therapy in the hope that something will work" approach. These were specific treatments, combined in concert and directed at specific problems. And while every case does not respond that quickly and favorably, a combination of specific therapies working in concert is more likely to produce the sweetest-sounding result.

■ Hitting the Mark

Some of the more interesting cases are those patients who have already tried practically everything without much success. Without reiterating the short-comings of nonspecific treatments, let me share an example that points out the difference between directed and nondirected, targeted and nontargeted.

A middle-aged woman came into the office with right-sided neck and upper back pain that periodically radiated into her right arm. Over the course of three years, she had tried physical therapy with exercise and strength training. It didn't help. She had also tried a massage therapist who actually did some deep tissue massage but missed "da shpot." Still no change. By the time she came to my office, this woman was almost resigned to the possibility that she would have to learn to live with the pain. I too was concerned, because the pain had now been there for an extended period and two of the three treatments I was about to recommend had already missed the mark.

The concert of therapies began with targeted deep massage, followed closely with spinal manipulation and extensive instruction in directed range of motion and stretching procedures to be done at home. Almost immediately, the patient noticed a significant difference in the application of the targeted massage and the stretching techniques. Right in the middle of the very first treatment, she said, "I had deep massage before, but nothing that ever felt like this." I am not suggesting the previous massage was improperly applied, but this patient's experience points out that unless the massage is targeted and specific, it is nothing more than an expensive, painful rubdown. When she returned for her second appointment, she said the directed stretching and range of motion had provided more relief than anything the physical therapy ever did. Although her prior physical therapy was most likely performed to the current standards, if it wasn't directed at the right joint structures and muscles, it too could easily have missed the mark. Within five visits, and in less than three weeks, this patient's three years of upper back pain and right arm tingling were completely gone. The concert of directed therapies was music to her ears—and to her back.

■ Putting It All Together

The last story is of a middle-aged man who was very active, playing tennis and golf several times a week. Occasionally he would come into the office for some weekend warrior muscle aches or pains, but he never had any prolonged or nonresolving complaints. One spring morning, he came in complaining of left-sided lower back pain radiating into his left buttock with numbness in his left upper thigh and leg. The regular concert of therapies was applied, and I told him to cut his activities in half, but after ten days there was only modest improvement. Four possible explanations for the slow response were running through my mind: I had missed the targets, he was doing too much in the way of activities, he was missing the targets with the stretching and exercise, or this was an acute herniated disc that was not going to respond to conservative treatment.

I recommended that he stop all activities and try to be more specific with his exercises, and I continued looking for other areas to target. Two more weeks had gone by, and there was still only minimal improvement. At this point, I had to consider the possibility of disc involvement, so I ordered an MRI, which revealed a herniated disc at a location corresponding to his symptoms. A surgical consultation was considered, but the patient decided to continue his follow-up with an orthopedist who prescribed physical therapy. Several weeks later, this man returned to my office with the symptoms completely unchanged. Because he had gotten some temporary relief from the targeted procedures in the past, he wanted to try them one more time before going under the knife. Having not made significant progress during the first attempt, I was reluctant to start over again, but at this point—with nothing to lose—we decided to give all three procedures another try.

Before we began, I wanted to be completely sure there was nothing we had missed the first time around. When I questioned him again about his activities, he confessed that he had never given them up. He also confessed that he had not actually done the home exercises during the first treatment period. This time, he promised to stop the tennis and golf, and he agreed to diligently perform the home stretching and range of motion exercises. Within one week he had made a 60 percent improvement, and by the end of the second week his symptoms were gone. Because there was no need to do a follow-up MRI, we will never know if the herniated disc changed, and quite frankly that doesn't really matter. What does matter is that given the proper combination of rest, exercise, and the concert of therapies, even people on the verge of spinal surgery may require only their own time, effort, and determination to make remarkable changes.

Think Back

Every doctor has the responsibility to bring out the best in each patient, and every patient has the responsibility to give the best effort possible. And while there is no formula for achieving your own successful outcome, education, persistence, and perseverance can never be compromised along the way. None of the stories in this chapter represent supernatural experiences or extraordinary superhuman efforts. These are people just like you who refused to give up and finally found a way to hit their mark.

Selected Bibliography

Aceves-Avila, F. J., R. Ferrari, and C. Ramos-Remus. 2004. New insights into cultural driven disorders. *Best Practice and Research: Clinical Rheumatology* 18 (2): 155–71.

Alao, A. O., and E. Faynberg. 2002. Chronic back pain successfully treated with supportive psychotherapy. *West African Journal of Medicine* 21 (2): 108–11.

Al-Obaidi, S. M., R. M. Nelson, S. Al-Awadhi, and N. Al-Shuwaie. 2000. The role of anticipation and fear of pain in the persistence of avoidance behavior in patients with chronic back pain. *Spine* 25 (9): 1126–31.

Assendelft, W. J., B. W. Koes, P. G. Knipschild, and L. M. Bouter. 1995. The relationship between methodological quality and conclusions in reviews of spinal manipulation. *Journal of the American Medical Association* 274 (24): 1942–48.

Atlas, S. J., and R. A. Deyo. 2001. Evaluating and managing acute low back pain in the primary care setting. *Journal of General Internal Medicine* 16 (2): 120–31.

Atlas, S. J., and E. Volinn. 1997. Classics from the spine literature revisited: A randomized trial of two versus seven days of recommended bed rest for acute low back pain. *Spine* 22 (20): 2331–37.

Bauman, A. E., B. Bellew, N. Owen, and P. Vita. 2001. Impact of an Australian mass media campaign targeting physical activity in 1998. *American Journal of Preventive Medicine* 21 (1): 41–47.

BenDabba, M., W. S. Torgerson, R. J. Boyd, E. G. Dawson, R. W. Hardy, J. T. Robertson, G. W. Sypert, C. Watts, and D. M. Long. 2002. Persistent low back pain and sciatica in the United States: Treatment outcomes. *Journal of Spinal Disorders Technology* 15 (1): 2–15.

Bolton, P., and A. Ware. 1988. Degenerative joint disease in the cervical spine of chiropractic patients. *Journal of the Australian Chiropractic Association* 18:51–54.

Boos, N., N. Semmer, A. Elfering, V. Schade, I. Gal, M. Zanetti, R. Kissling, N. Buchegger, J. Hodler, and C. J. Main. 2000. Natural history of individuals with asymptomatic disc abnormalities in magnetic resonance imaging: Predictors of low back pain–related medical consultation and work incapacity. *Spine* 25 (12): 1484–92.

Bronfort, G. 1999. Spinal manipulation: Current state of research and its indications. *Neurology Clinician* 17 (1): 91–111.

Bronfort, G., R. Evans, B. Nelson, P. D. Aker, C. H. Goldsmith, and H. Vernon. 2001. A randomized clinical trial of exercise and spinal manipulation for patients with chronic neck pain. *Spine* 26 (7): 788–99.

Bronfort, G., M. Haas, R. L. Evans, and L. M. Bouter. 2004. Efficacy of spinal manipulation and mobilization for low back pain and neck pain: A systematic review and best evidence synthesis. *Spine Journal* 4 (3): 335–56.

Burton, A. K., K. M. Tillotson, C. J. Main, and S. Hollis. 1995. Psychosocial predictors of outcome in acute and subchronic low back trouble. *Spine* 20 (6): 722–28.

Burton, A. K., G. Waddell, K. M. Tillotson, and N. Summerton. 1999. Information and advice to patients with back pain can have a positive effect: A randomized controlled trial of a novel educational booklet in primary care. *Spine* 24 (23): 2484–91.

Butterman, G. R. 2004. Treatment of lumbar disc herniation: Epidural steroid injection compared with discectomy. A prospective randomized study. *Journal of Bone and Joint Surgery* 86-A (4): 670–79.

Carey, T. S., J. Garrett, A. Jackman, C. McLaughlin, J. Fryer, and D. R. Smucker. 1995. The outcomes and cost of care for acute low back pain among patients seen by primary care practitioners, chiropractors, and orthopedic surgeons. *New England Journal of Medicine* 333 (14): 913–17.

Cherkin, D. C., D. Eisenberg, K. J. Sherman, W. Barlow, T. J. Kaptchuk, J. Street, and R. A. Deyo. 2001. Randomized trial comparing traditional Chinese medical acupuncture, therapeutic massage, and self-care education for low back pain. *Archives of Internal Medicine* 161 (8): 1081–88.

Cohen, I., and J. Rainville. 2002. Aggressive exercise as treatment for chronic low back pain. *Sports Medicine* 32 (1): 75–82.

Cooper, J. E., R. B. Tate, A. Yassi, and J. Khokhar. 1996. Effect of an early intervention program on the relationship between subjective pain and disability measures in nurses with low back injury. *Spine* 21 (20): 2329–36.

Coulter, I. D. 1996. Efficacy and risk of chiropractic manipulation: What does the evidence suggest? *Integrative Medicine* 1:61–66.

Ernst, E., and M. H. Pittler. 1999. Experts' opinions on complementary/alternative therapies for low back pain. *Journal of Manipulative Therapeutics* 22 (2): 87–90.

Evans, R. W. 1992. Some observations on whiplash injuries. *Neurology Clinician* 10 (4): 975–97.

Fitz-Ritzon, D. 1995. Phasic exercises for cervical rehabilitation after whiplash trauma. *Journal of Manipulative Therapeutics* 18 (1): 21–24.

Fritz, J. M., S. Z. George, and A. Delitto. 2001. The role of fear avoidance beliefs in acute low back pain: Relationships with current and future disability and work status. *Pain* 94 (1): 7–15.

Frost, H., S. E. Lamb, H. A. Doll, P. T. Carver, and S. Stuart-Brown. 2004. Randomized controlled trial of physiotherapy compared with advise for low back pain. *British Medical Journal* 329 (7468): 708.

Frost, H., S. E. Lamb, J. A. Moffett, J. C. Fairbank, and J. S. Moser. 1998. A fitness program for patients with chronic low back pain: Two year follow-up of a randomized controlled trial. *Pain* 75 (2–3): 273–79.

Gay, R. 1993. The curve of the cervical spine: Variations and significance. *Journal of Manipulative and Physiological Therapeutics* 16 (9): 591–94.

Geisser, M. E., A. J. Haig, A. S. Wallbom, and E. A. Wiggert. 2004. Pain-related fear, lumbar flexion, and dynamic EMG among persons with chronic musculoskeletal low back pain. *Clinical Journal of Pain* 20 (2): 61–69.

Gore, D. R., S. B. Sepic, G. M. Gardner, and M. P. Murray. 1987. Neck pain: A long-term follow-up of 205 patients. *Spine* 12 (1): 1–5.

Hagen, K. B., H. H. Holte, K. Tambs, and T. Bjerkedal. 2000. Socioeconomic factors and disability retirement from back pain: A 1983–1993 population-based prospective study in Norway. *Spine* 25 (19): 2480–87.

Hanton, W. P., S. L. Olson, N. L. Butts, and A. L. Nowicki. 2000. Effective-ness of a home program of ischemic pressure followed by sustained stretch for treatment of myofascial trigger points. *Physiological Therapeutics* 81 (4): 1059–60.

Hayden, J. A., M. W. van Tulder, and G. Tomlinson. 2005. Systematic review: Strategies for using exercise therapy to improve outcomes in chronic low back pain. *Annals of Internal Medicine* 142 (9): 776–85.

Helliwell, P. S., P. F. Evans, and V. Wright. 1994. The straight cervical spine: Does it indicate spasm? *Journal of Bone and Joint Surgery* 76 (1): 103–6.

Hertzman-Miller, R. P., H. Morganstern, E. L. Hurwitz, F. Yu, A. H. Adams, P. Harber, and G. F. Kominski. 2002. Comparing the satisfaction of low back pain patients randomized to receive medical or chiropractic care: Results from the UCLA low back pain study. *American Journal of Public Health* 92 (10): 1628–33.

Hicks, G. S., D. N. Duddleston, L. D. Russell, H. E. Holman, J. M. Shepard, and C. A. Brown. 2002. Low back pain. *American Journal of Medical Science* 324 (4): 207–11.

Hoving, J. L., B. W. Koes, H. C. de Vet, D. A. van der Windt, W. J. Assendelft, H. van Mameren, W. L. Deville, J. J. Pool, R. J. Scholton, and L. M. Bouter. 2002. Manual therapy, physical therapy, or continued care by a general practitioner for patients with neck pain: A randomized controlled trial. *Annals of Internal Medicine* 136 (10): 713–22.

Hurwitz, E. L., P. D. Aker, A. H. Adams, W. C. Meeker, and P. G. Shekelle. 1996. Manipulation and mobilization of the cervical spine: A systematic review of the literature. *Spine* 21 (15): 1759–60.

Jordan, A., T. Bendix, H. Nielsen, F. R. Hansen, D. Host, and A. Winkel. 1998. Intensive training, physiotherapy, or manipulation for patients with chronic neck pain: A prospective single-blinded, randomized clinical trial. *Spine* 23 (3): 311–18.

Karlsborg, M., A. Smed, H. Jespersen, S. Stephensen, M. Cortsen, P. Jennum, M. Herning, E. Korfitsen, and L. Werdelin. 1997. A prospective study of thirty-nine patients with whiplash injury. *Acta Neurology Scandinavia* 95 (2): 65–72.

Kendall, N. A. 1999. Psychological approaches to the prevention of chronic pain: The low back paradigm. *Bailliere's Best Practice and Research: Clinical Rheumatology* 13 (3): 545–54.

Khot, A., M. Bowditch, J. Powell, and D. Sharp. 2004. The use of interdiscal steroid therapy for lumbar spinal discogenic pain: A randomized controlled study. *Spine* 29 (8): 833–36.

Kopec, J. A., E. C. Sayre, and J. M. Esdaile. 2004. Predictors of back pain in a general population cohort. *Spine* 29 (1): 70–77.

Krause, N., L. K. Dasinger, L. J. Deegan, L. Randolph, and R. J. Brand. 2001. Psychosocial job factors and return-to-work after compensated low back injury: A disability phase–specific analysis. *American Journal of Industrial Medicine* 40 (4): 374–92.

Leclaire, R., L. Fortin, R. Lambert, Y. M. Bergeron, and M. Rossignol. 2001. Radiofrequency facet joint denervation in the treatment of low back pain: A placebo-controlled clinical trial to assess efficacy. *Spine* 26 (13): 1411–16.

Leclerc, A., I. Neidhammer, M. F. Landre, A. Ozguler, P. Etore, and F. Pietre-Taleb. 1999. One year predictive factors for various aspects of neck disorders. *Spine* 24 (14): 1455–62.

Licht, P. B., H. W. Christensen, and P. F. Hoilund-Carlsen. 2003. Is cervical spine manipulation dangerous? *Journal of Manipulative and Physiological Therapeutics* 26 (1): 48–52.

Linton, S. J., and T. Andersson. 2000. Can chronic disability be prevented? A randomized trial of cognitive-behavior intervention and two forms of information for patients with spinal pain. *Spine* 25 (21): 2825–31.

Linton, S. J., and M. Ryberg. 2001. A cognitive behavioral group intervention as prevention for persistent neck and back pain in a non-patient population: A randomized controlled trial. *Pain* 90 (1): 83–90.

Long, D. W., M. BenDabba, W. S. Torgerson, R. J. Boyd, E. G. Dawson, R. W. Hardy, J. T. Robertson, G. W. Sypert, and C. Watts. 1996. Persistent low back pain and sciatica in the United States: Pain characteristics. *Journal of Spinal Disorders* 9 (1): 40–58.

Mannion, A. F., M. Muntener, S. Taimela, and J. Dvorak. 1999. A randomized clinical trial of three active therapies for chronic low back pain. *Spine* 24 (23): 2435–48.

———. 2001. Comparison of three active therapies for chronic low back pain: Results of a randomized clinical trial with one-year follow-up. *Rheumatology* 40 (7): 772–78.

Matsumoto, M., K. Chiba, M. Ishikawa, H. Maruiwa, Y. Fujimura, and Y. Toyama. 2001. Relationships between outcomes of conservative treatment and magnetic resonance imaging findings in patients with mild cervical myelopathy caused by soft disc herniations. *Spine* 26 (14): 1592–98.

Matsumoto, M., Y. Fujimura, N. Suzuki, Y. Toyama, and H. Shiga. 1998. Cervical curvature in acute whiplash injuries: Prospective comparative study with asymptomatic subjects. *Injury* 29 (10): 775–78.

McPhillips-Tangum, C. A., D. C. Cherkin, L. A. Rhodes, and C. Markham. 1998. Reasons for repeated medical visits among patients with chronic back pain. *Journal of General Internal Medicine* 13 (5): 289–95.

Meade, T. W., S. Dyer, W. Browne, and A. O. Frank. 1995. Randomized comparison of chiropractic and hospital outpatient management for low back pain: Results from extended follow-up. *British Medical Journal* 311 (7015): 1301–2.

Michel, A., T. Kohlmann, and H. Raspe. 1997. The association between clinical findings on physical examination and self-reported severity in back pain. *Spine* 22 (3): 303–4.

Mikeladze, G., R. Espinal, R. Finnegan, J. Routon, and D. Martin. 2003. Pulsed radiofrequency application in treatment of chronic zygapophyseal joint pain. *Spine Journal* 3 (5): 360–62.

Moore, J. E., M. Von Korff, D. Cherkin, K. Saunders, and K. Lorig. 2000. A randomized trial of a cognitive behavioral program for enhancing back pain self-care in a primary care setting. *Pain* 88 (2): 145–53.

Ong, A., J. Anderson, and J. Roche. 2003. A pilot study of the prevalence of lumbar disc degeneration in elite athletes with lower back pain at the Sydney 2000 Olympic games. *British Journal of Sports Medicine* 37 (3): 263–66.

Picavet, H. S., J. W. Vlaeyen, and J. S. Schouten. 2002. Pain catastrophizing and kinesiophobia: Predictors of chronic pain. *American Journal of Epidemiology* 156 (11): 1028–34.

Power, C., J. Frank, C. Hertzman, G. Schierhout, and L. Li. 2001. Predictors of low back pain onset in a prospective British study. *American Journal of Public Health* 91 (10): 1671–78.

Preyde, M. 2000. Effectiveness of massage therapy for subacute low back pain: A randomized controlled study. *Canadian Medical Association Journal* 162 (13): 1815–20.

Reis, S. D., D. Hermoni, J. M. Borkan, A. Biderman, C. Tabenkin, and A. Porat. 1999. A new look at low back complaints in primary care. *Journal of Family Practice* 48 (4): 299–303.

Rose, M. J., J. P. Reilly, B. Pennie, K. Bowen-Jones, I. M. Stanley, and P. D. Slade. 1997. Chronic low back pain rehabilitation programs: A study of the optimum duration of treatment and a comparison of group and individual therapy. *Spine* 22 (19): 2246–51.

Rust, M. S., and W. C. Olivero. 1999. Far lateral disc herniations: The results of conservative management. *Journal of Spinal Disorders* 12 (2): 138–40.

Schrader, H., D. Obelieniene, G. Bovim, D. Surkiene, D. Mickeviciene, I. Miseviciene, and T. Sand. 1999. Natural evolution of late whiplash syndrome outside the medicolegal context. *Lancet* 347 (9010): 1207–11.

Schultz, I. Z., J. M. Crook, J. Berkowitz, G. R. Meloche, R. Milner, O. A. Zuberbier, and W. Meloche. 2002. Biopsychosocial multivariate predictive model of occupational low back disability. *Spine* 27 (23): 2720–25.

Seferlis, T., G. Nemeth, A. M. Carlsson, and P. Gillstrom. 1998. Conservative treatment in patients sick-listed for acute low-back pain: A prospective randomised study with twelve months' follow-up. *European Spine Journal* 7 (6): 461–70.

Skargen, E. I., and B. E. Oberg. 1998. Predictive factors for one year outcome of low back and neck pain in patients treated in primary care: Comparison between the treatment strategies for chiropractic and physiotherapy. *Pain* 77 (2): 201–7.

Skargen, E. I., B. E. Oberg, P. G. Carlsson, and M. Gade. 1997. Cost and effectiveness analysis of chiropractic and physiotherapy treatment for low back and neck pain: Six-month follow-up. *Spine* 22 (18): 2167–77.

Smith, D., N. McMurray, and P. Disler. 2002. Early intervention for acute back injury: Can we finally develop an evidence-based approach? *Clinical Rehabilitation* 16 (1): 1–11.

Spruit, M., and W. C. Jacobs. 2002. Pain and function after intradiscal electrothermal treatment (IDET) for symptomatic lumbar disc degeneration. *European Spine Journal* 11 (6): 589–93.

Staerkle, R., A. F. Mannion, A. Elfering, A. Junge, N. K. Semmer, N. Jacobshagen, D. Grob, J. Dvorak, and N. Boos. 2004. Longitudinal validation of the Fear-Avoidance Beliefs Questionnaire (FABQ) in a Swiss-German sample of low back pain patients. *European Spine Journal* 13 (4): 332–40.

Stevinson, C., and E. Ernst. 2002. Risks associated with spinal manipulation. *American Journal of Medicine* 112 (7): 566–71.

Suissa, S. 2003. Risk factors of poor prognosis after whiplash injury. *Pain Management* 8 (2): 69–75.

Symonds, T. L., A. K. Burton, K. M. Tillotson, and C. J. Main. 1996. Do attitudes and beliefs influence work loss due to low back trouble? *Occupational Medicine* 46 (1): 25–32.

Thomas, E., A. J. Silman, P. R. Croft, A. C. Papageorgiou, M. I. Jayson, and G. J. Macfarlane. 1999. Predicting who develops chronic low back pain in primary care: A prospective study. *British Medical Journal* 318 (7199): 1662–67.

Torstensen, T. A., A. E. Ljunggren, H. D. Meen, E. Odland, P. Mowinckel, and S. Geijerstam. 1998. Efficiency and costs of medical exercise therapy, conventional physiotherapy, and self exercise in patients with chronic low back pain. *Spine* 23 (23): 2616–24.

van Tulder, M. W., A. Malmivaara, R. Esmail, and B. W. Koes. 2000. Exercise therapy for low back pain. *Cochrane Database Systematic Review* 2:CD000335.

Verbeek, J., M. J. Sengers, L. Riemens, and J. Haafkens. 2004. Patient expectations of treatment for low back pain: A systematic review of qualitative and quantitative studies. *Spine* 29 (20): 2309–18.

Von Korff, M., J. E. Moore, K. Lorig, D. C. Cherkin, K. Saunders, V. M. Gonzalez, D. Laurent, C. Rutter, and F. Comite. 1998. A randomized trial of lay person–led self-management group intervention for back pain patients in primary care. *Spine* 23 (23): 2608–15.

References Cited

Agency for Health Care Policy and Research. 1994. *Clinical Practice Guideline* 14: 68.

Atlas, S. J., and R. A. Nardin. 2003. Evaluation and treatment of low back pain: An evidence-based approach to clinical care. *Muscle and Nerve* 27 (3): 265–84.

Bartleson, J. D. 2001. Low back pain. *Current Treatment Options in Neurology* 3 (2): 159–68.

Boden, S. D., D. O. Davis, T. S. Dina, N. J. Patronas, and S. W. Wiesel. 1990. Abnormal magnetic resonance scans of the lumbar spine in asymptomatic subjects. A prospective investigation. *Journal of Bone and Joint Surgery* 72 (3): 403–8.

Boden, S. D., P. R. McCowin, D. O. Davis, T. S. Dina, A. S. Mark, and S. Wiesel. 1990. Abnormal magnetic resonance scans of the cervical spine in asymptomatic subjects. A prospective investigation. *Journal of Bone and Joint Surgery* 72 (8): 1178–84.

Borchgrevink, G. E., A. Kaasa, D. McDonagh, T. Stiles, O. Haraldseth, and I. Lereim. 1998. Acute treatment of whiplash neck sprain injuries. *Spine* 23 (1): 25–31.

Borenstein, D. G., J. W. O'Mara, S. D. Boden, W. C. Lauerman, A. Jacobson, C. Platenberg, D. Schellinger, and S. W. Wiesel. 2001. The value of magnetic resonance imaging of the lumbar spine to predict low-back pain in asymptomatic subjects. *Journal of Bone and Joint Surgery* 83-A (9): 1306–11.

Buchbinder, R., D. Jolley, and M. Wyatt. 2001. Population based intervention to change back pain beliefs and disability: Three part evaluation. *British Medical Journal* 322 (7301): 1516–20.

Buer, N., and S. J. Linton. 2002. Fear-avoidance beliefs and catastrophizing: Occurrence and risk factor in back pain ADL in the general population. *Pain* 99 (3): 485–91.

Burton, A. K., T. D. McClune, R. D. Clarke, and C. J. Main. 2004. Long-term follow-up of patients with low back pain attending for manipulative care: Outcomes and predictors. *Manual Therapy* 9 (1): 30–35.

Carey, T. S., J. M. Garrett, A. Jackman, and N. Hadler. 1999. Recurrence and care seeking after acute back injury: Results of a long-term follow-up study. *Medical Care* 37 (2): 157–64.

Carragee, E. J., T. F. Alamin, J. L. Miller, and J. M. Carragee. 2005. Discographic, MRI, and psychological determinants of low back pain disability and remission: A prospective study in subjects with benign persistent back pain. *Spine Journal* 5 (1): 24–35.

Carragee, E. J., B. Barcohana, T. Alamin, and E. van den Haak. 2004. Prospective controlled study of the development of lower back pain in previously asymptomatic subjects undergoing experimental discography. *Spine* 29 (10): 1112–17.

Cherkin, D. C., R. A. Deyo, M. Battie, J. Street, and W. Barlow. 1998. A comparison of physical therapy, chiropractic manipulation, and provision of an educational booklet for the treatment of patients with low back pain. *New England Journal of Medicine* 339 (15): 1021–29.

Cherkin, D. C., K. J. Sherman, R. A. Deyo, and P. G. Shekelle. 2003. A review of the evidence for the effectiveness, safety, and cost of acupuncture, massage therapy, and spinal manipulation for back pain. *Annals of Internal Medicine* 138 (11): 898–906.

Croft, P. R., G. J. Macfarlane, A. C. Papageorgiou, E. Thomas, and A. J. Silman. 1998. Outcome of low back pain in general practice: A prospective study. *British Medical Journal* 316 (7141): 1356–59.

Davis, T. T., R. B. Delamarter, P. Sra, and T. B. Goldstein. 2004. The IDET procedure for chronic discogenic low back pain. *Spine* 29 (7): 752–56.

Delport, E. G., A. R. Cucuzzella, J. K. Marley, C. M. Pruitt, and J. R. Fisher. 2004. Treatment for lumbar spinal stenosis with epidural steroid injections: A retrospective outcome study. *Archives of Physical Medicine and Rehabilitation* 85 (3): 479–84.

Dionne, C. E., M. Von Korff, T. D. Koepsell, R. A. Deyo, W. E. Barlow, and H. Checkoway. 2001. Formal education and back pain: A review. *Journal of Epidemiology in Community Health* 55 (7): 455–68.

Edwards, R., E. Augustson, and R. Fillingim. 2003. Differential relationships between anxiety and treatment-associated pain reduction among male and female chronic pain patients. *Clinical Journal of Pain* 19 (4): 208–16.

Ehrlich, G. E. 2003a. Back pain. *Journal of Rheumatology* 67:26–31.

Ehrlich, G. E. 2003b. Low back pain. *Bulletin of the World Health Organization* 81 (9): 671–76.

Eisenberg, D. M., R. B. Davis, S. L. Ettner, S. Appel, S. Wilkey, M. Van Rompay, and R. C. Kessler. 1998. Trends in alternative medicine use in the United States, 1990–1997: Results of a follow-up national survey. *Journal of the American Medical Association* 280:1569–1575.

Ellenberg, M., M. Ross, J. Honet, M. Schwartz, G. Chodoroff, and S. Enohs. 1983. Prospective evaluation of the course of disc herniations in patients with proven radiculopathy. *Archives of Medical Rehabilitation* 74:3–8.

Ferrari, R., C. Constantoyannis, and N. Papadakis. 2003. Laypersons' expectations of the sequelae of whiplash injury: A cross-cultural comparative study between Canada and Greece. *Medical Science Monitor* 9 (3): CR120–24.

Ferrari, R., A. S. Russell, and M. Richter. 2001. Epidemiology of whiplash injuries: An international dilemma. *Der Orthopäde* 30 (8): 551–58.

Frymoyer, J. W., and W. L. Cats-Baril. 1991. An overview of the incidences and costs of low back pain. *Orthopedic Clinics of North America* 22 (2): 263–71.

Gatchel, R. J., P. B. Polatin, C. Noe, M. Gardea, C. Pulliam, and J. Thompson. 2003. Treatment- and cost-effectiveness of early intervention for acute low-back pain patients: A one-year prospective study. *Journal of Occupational Rehabilitation* 13 (1): 1–9.

Gillan, M. G., F. J. Gilbert, J. E. Andrew, A. M. Grant, D. Wardlaw, N. W. Valentine, and A. C. Gregori. 2001. Influence of imaging on clinical decision making in the treatment of lower back pain. *Radiology* 220 (2): 393–99.

Georgetown University Center on an Aging Society. 2003. *Chronic Back Pain*. Challenges for the twenty-first century: Chronic and disabling conditions, Date Profile no. 8. Washington, DC: Georgetown University.

Glenton, C. 2003. Chronic back pain sufferers: Striving for the sick role. *Social Science Medicine* 57 (11): 2243–52.

Grover, F., and S. L. Pereira. 2003. Is MRI useful for evaluation of acute low back pain? *Journal of Family Practice* 52 (3): 231–32.

Hagen, E. M., H. R. Eriksen, and H. Ursin. 2000. Does early intervention with a light mobilization program reduce long-term sick leave for low back pain? *Spine* 25 (15): 1973–76.

Hernandez-Reif, M., T. Field, J. Krasnegor, and H. Theakston. 2001. Lower back pain is reduced and range of motion is increased after massage therapy. *International Journal of Neuroscience* 106 (3–4): 131–34.

Hurwitz, E. L., H. Morganstern, P. Harber, G. F. Kominski, T. R. Berlin, F. Yu, and A. H. Adams. 2002. A randomized trial of medical care with and without physical therapy and chiropractic care with and without physical modalities for patients with low back pain. *Spine* 27 (20): 2193–204.

Indahl, A. 2004. Low back pain: Diagnosis, treatment, and prognosis. *Scandinavian Journal of Rheumatology* 33 (4): 199–209.

Jarvik, J. G., W. Hollingworth, P. J. Heagerty, D. R. IIaynor, E. J. Boyko, and R. A. Deyo. 2005. Three-year incidence of low back pain in an initially asymptomatic cohort: Clinical and imaging risk factors. *Spine* 30 (13): 1541–48.

Jensen, M., M. Brant-Zawadzki, N. Obuchowski, M. Modic, D. Malkasian, and J. Ross. 1994. Magnetic resonance imaging of the lumbar spine in people without back pain. *New England Journal of Medicine* 331 (2): 69–73.

Kalauokalani, D., D. C. Cherkin, K. J. Sherman, T. D. Koepsell, and R. A. Deyo. 2001. Lessons from a trial of acupuncture and massage for low back pain: Patient expectations and treatment effects. *Spine* 26 (13): 1418–24.

Kauppila, L. I., S. Eustace, D. P. Kiel, D. T. Felson, and A. M. Wright. 1998. Degenerative displacement of lumbar vertebrae. A twenty-five year follow-up study in Framingham. *Spine* 23 (17): 1868–73.

Lestini, W. F., and S. Wiesel. 1989. Acute cervical herniation. *Clinical Orthopedics* 239:69–93.

Linton, S. J. 2000. A review of psychological risk factors in back and neck pain. *Spine* 25 (9): 1148–56.

Linton, S. J., and M. W. van Tulder. 2001. Preventive interventions for neck and back pain problems: What is the evidence? *Spine* 26 (7): 778–87.

Lively, M. W. 2002. Sports medicine approach to low back pain. *Southern Medical Journal* 95 (6): 642–46.

Livingston, M. 1992. Whiplash injury: Misconceptions and remedies. *Australian Family Physician* 21 (11): 1642–43.

Long, A., R. Donelson, and T. Fung. 2004. Does it matter which exercise? A randomized control trial of exercise for low back pain. *Spine* 29 (33): 2593–602.

Maigne, J., B. Rime, and B. Delignet. 1992. Computed tomographic follow-up of forty-eight cases of nonoperatively treated lumbar intervertebral disc herniation. *Spine* 17 (9): 1071–74.

Manek, N. J., and A. J. MacGregor. 2005. Epidemiology of back disorders: Prevalence, risk factors, and prognosis. *Current Opinion in Rheumatology* 17 (2): 134–40.

McKinney, L. A. 1989. Early mobilization and outcome in acute sprains of the neck. *British Medical Journal* 299 (6706): 1006–8.

Miller, J. A., C. Schmatz, and A. B. Schultz. 1988. Lumbar disc degeneration: Correlation with age, sex, and spine level in 600 autopsy specimens. *Spine* 13 (2): 173–78.

Moffett, J. K., D. Torgerson, S. Bell-Syer, D. Jackson, H. Llewlyn-Phillips, A. Farrin, and J. Barber. 1999. Randomized controlled trial of exercise for low back pain: Clinical outcomes, costs, and preferences. *British Medical Journal* 319 (7205): 279–83.

Mootz, R. D., D. T. Hansen, T. A. Souza, J. J. Triano, and B. C. Wiese. 2000. Application of incremental change strategies in chiropractic and multidisciplinary settings for quality improvement. *Quality Managed Health Care* 8 (3): 42–64.

Murrie, V. L., A. K. Dixon, W. Hollingworth, H. Wilson, and T. A. Doyle. 2003. Lumbar lordosis: Study of patients with and without low back pain. *Clinical Anatomy* 16 (2): 144–47.

Niemisto, L., E. Kalso, A. Malmivaara, S. Seitsalo, and H. Hurri. 2003. Radiofrequency denervation for neck and back pain: A systematic review within the framework of the Cochrane collaboration back review group. *Spine* 28 (16): 1877–88.

Obelieniene, D., H. Schrader, G. Bovim, I. Miseviciene, and T. Sand. 1999. Pain after whiplash: A prospective controlled inception cohort study. *Journal of Neurology and Neurosurgical Psychiatry* 66 (3): 279–83.

Partheni, M., C. Constantoyannis, R. Ferrari, G. Nikiforidis, S. Voulgaris, and N. Papadakis. 2000. A prospective cohort study of the outcome of acute whiplash injury in Greece. *Clinical Experimental Rheumatology* 18 (1): 67–70.

Pettersson, K., C. Hildingsson, G. Toolanen, M. Fagerlund, and J. Bjornebrink. 1997. Disc pathology after whiplash injury: A prospective magnetic resonance imaging and clinical investigation. *Spine* 22 (3): 283–87.

Pincus, T., A. K. Burton, S. Vogel, and A. P. Field. 2002. A systematic review of psychological factors as predictors of chronicity/disability in prospective cohorts of low back pain. *Spine* 27 (5): E109–20.

Reeser, J. C., S. M. Wiegmann, N. Hoover, N. Oldridge, D. Phillips, T. Bjelland, L. Scarpinato, W. Treacy, C. P. Helstad, and J. Stoll. 2001. Treatment of acute low back pain in Wisconsin: Results of the State Medical Society's medical outcomes research project. *Wisconsin Medical Journal* 100 (8): 35–42.

Rizzo, J. A., T. A. Abbott, and M. L. Berger. 1998. The labor productivity effects of chronic backache in the United States. *Medical Care* 36 (10): 1471–88.

Rosenfeld, M., R. Gunnarsson, and P. Borenstein. 2000. Early intervention in whiplash-associated disorders: A comparison of two treatment protocols. *Spine* 25 (14): 1782–87.

Savage, R. A., G. H. Whitehouse, and N. Roberts. 1997. The relationship between the magnetic resonance imaging appearance of the lumbar spine and low back pain, age, and occupation in males. *European Spine Journal* 6 (2): 106–14.

Soderlund, A., and P. Lindberg. 2003. Whiplash-associated disorders: Predicting disability from a process-oriented perspective of coping. *Clinical Rehabilitation* 17 (1): 101–7.

van den Hoogen, H. J., B. W. Koes, W. Deville, J. T. van Eijk, and L. M. Bouter. 1997. The prognosis of low back pain in general practice. *Spine* 22 (13): 1515–21.

van Tulder, M. W., R. J. Scholten, B. W. Koes, and R. A. Deyo. 2000. Nonsteroidal anti-inflammatory drugs for low back pain: A systematic review within the framework of the Cochrane collaboration back review group. *Spine* 25 (19): 2501–13.

Vlaeyen, J. W., and S. J. Linton. 2000. Fear-avoidance and its consequences in chronic musculoskeletal pain: A state of the art. *Pain* 85 (3): 317–32.

Wand, B. M., C. Bird, J. H. McAuley, C. J. Dore, M. MacDowell, and L. H. De Souza. 2004. Early intervention for the management of acute low back pain: A single-blind randomized controlled trial of biopsychosocial education, manual therapy, and exercise. *Spine* 29 (21): 2350–56.

Wiesel, S., N. Tsourmas, H. Feffer, C. Citrin, and N. Patronas. 1984. A study of computer-assisted tomography. I. The incidence of positive CAT scans in an asymptomatic group of patients. *Spine* 9 (6): 549–51.

Zanni, G., and J. Wick. 2003. Low back pain: Eliminating myths and elucidating realities. *Journal of the American Pharmaceutical Association* 43 (3): 357–62.

Gerald M. Silverman, DC, is a 1978 graduate of Palmer College of Chiropractic and a board-certified chiropractic physician in private practice in Hauppauge, NY. He interned in the Department of Radiology at Palmer College and is a diplomate of the National Board of Chiropractic Examiners. He has completed postgraduate study at New York Chiropractic College in applied spinal disability and impairment rating and received a degree in applied chiropractic sciences from Life Chiropractic College West. He has lectured at professional conferences and symposia.

Some Other New Harbinger Titles

Solid to the Core, Item 4305 $14.95

Staying Focused in the Age of Distraction, Item 433X $16.95

Living Beyond Your Pain, Item 4097 $19.95

Fibromyalgia & Chronic Fatigue Syndrome, Item 4593 $14.95

Your Miraculous Back, Item 4526 $18.95

TriEnergetics, Item 4453 $15.95

Emotional Fitness for Couples, Item 4399 $14.95

The MS Workbook, Item 3902 $19.95

Depression & Your Thyroid, Item 4062 $15.95

The Eating Wisely for Hormonal Balance Journal, Item 3945 $15.95

Healing Adult Acne, Item 4151 $15.95

The Memory Doctor, Item 3708 $11.95

The Emotional Wellness Way to Cardiac Health, Item 3740 $16.95

The Cyclothymia Workbook, Item 383X $18.95

The Matrix Repatterning Program for Pain Relief, Item 3910 $18.95

Transforming Stress, Item 397X $10.95

Eating Mindfully, Item 3503 $13.95

Living with RSDS, Item 3554 $16.95

The Ten Hidden Barriers to Weight Loss, Item 3244 $11.95

The Sjogren's Syndrome Survival Guide, Item 3562 $15.95

Stop Feeling Tired, Item 3139 $14.95

Responsible Drinking, Item 2949 $19.95

The Mitral Valve Prolapse/Dysautonomia Survival Guide, Item 3031 $14.95

The Vulvodynia Survival Guide, Item 2914 $16.95

The Multifidus Back Pain Solution, Item 2787 $12.95

Move Your Body, Tone Your Mood, Item 2752 $17.95

The Trigger Point Therapy Workbook, Item 2507 $19.95

Fibromyalgia and Chronic Myofascial Pain Syndrome, second edition, Item 2388 $19.95

Call **toll free, 1-800-748-6273,** or log on to our online bookstore at **www.newharbinger.com** to order. Have your Visa or Mastercard number ready. Or send a check for the titles you want to New Harbinger Publications, Inc., 5674 Shattuck Ave., Oakland, CA 94609. Include $4.50 for the first book and 75¢ for each additional book, to cover shipping and handling. (California residents please include appropriate sales tax.) Allow two to five weeks for delivery.

Prices subject to change without notice.